The Pink Mountain

By Cindy Needham

The Pink Mountain

Copyright @ 2020 Cindy Needham

www.thrivetheclimb.com

Published by Follow It Thru Publishing

www.heatherandrews.press

www.getyouvisible.com

www.followitthrupublishing.com

Print ISBN:
978-1-989848-03-6

eBook ISBN:
978-1-989848-04-3

Dedication

This book is dedicated to…

My late birth mom, Linda (Carriere) Robinson, whose own journey ended on the Pink Mountain, after a long and courageous battle;

and to

My late parents, Norma and Barrie Needham—I know you are smiling down on me;

and to

My partner and soul mate, Cheryl Stephenson, who has been along side of me every step of this Pink Mountain.

Gratitude

I believe that a great climber is only as great as the team around her. I want to express my gratitude to the following people, whose unconditional love and support was a breath of fresh air, adding to my strength as I climbed the Pink Mountain.

My Kentwood Family: Thank you, **Tanya Snelson, Nolana Nichols, Kim Sinclair, Shanna Hutchison,** and **Alison Kelly.** You made a huge difference in helping us adapt to the many surprises that cancer treatment brought. You are all not just my neighbors, you are my family.

My friend **Susan Becker.** I felt your love and support from afar. After 27 years of friendship, I know you were emotionally invested in my journey. Cheers to many more years my beautiful friend!

Gail Frasz, who has become my mother figure. Having a mama bear standing behind me has been comforting in more ways than I can count. Thank you for making room for me in your heart!

Acknowledgements

This book would still be a dream, floating around in my mind, if it wasn't for the series of events and people that were important catalysts in bringing this dream to life. I would like to thank the following people…

My network of **awesome friends,** who took the time to read and respond to my emails, Facebook updates and blogs throughout my cancer journey. Your encouraging words sparked the idea, that I could write a book that would help other women going through this hard and complex journey.

In October 2018, my friend **Karen Rowe** was offering a six-week writing course. I decided that if I wanted to get the thoughts in my head into words on paper, investing in Karen's course was what I needed to do. While it took me longer than six weeks to write my draft, without this course, I never would have gotten my feet moving. Thank you, Karen.

Thank you, **Christine Maul** for introducing me to the incredible **Tammy Jensen,** (an author herself, with a keen editing eye) who read my manuscript and gave me the courage to stretch my wings and fly.

I want to thank **Heather Andrews** and her team at **Get You Visible Publishing** for helping me take my message from a manuscript, to the book you are now holding and reading. A big shout out to **Lorraine Shulba** for the incredible artwork on the cover, and to **Daphne Street** for her excellent job on editing.

Thank you, **Andrea Carter** for believing in me and the importance of the message I am delivering to the world. Words can't adequately describe the insight, passion and energy you have brought to the finishing touches of this book. Because of you and your wisdom, The Pink Mountain will now make it into the hands of the countless women who need it.

To my partner of twenty years, **Cheryl Stephenson**. Thank you for being my biggest fan. This book would not have happened without you, or all of your "backstage" support. You worked endlessly making sure life around us kept moving forward when my head was down and focused on writing. When I did come up for air, you always greeted me with a smile and wanted to know how my book was going. When I did need help, you would often stop what you were doing and work with me, to make sense of my fragmented thoughts. Your time, patience, encouragement and support, helped to make my dream a reality. You may have been "backstage" on this book, but in life, I am truly blessed to be walking beside you. Thank you, for being you!

Table of Contents

FOREWORD

A Spiritual Journey of Hope

and Empowerment

by Daphne Taylor Street

I had the honor of editing Cindy Needham's manuscript, The Pink Mountain, and I suppose that also means that I was one of the first to read this work. As an editor, it also means that I had the privilege to take a deep-dive into the content, to delve into the stories, lessons, and the experience that Cindy is offering to the world, and I found myself personally affected by it. I have been writing and editing professionally for about 20 years, and one of my gifts that I give and receive, equally, is this immersion process with others' stories. Working on The Pink Mountain was no exception, but it had a profound impact on me personally—one that I shared with Cindy, who then asked me to write this foreword.

When you read The Pink Mountain, you will be guided on a journey through Cindy's experience as a breast cancer survivor, from diagnosis through treatment, and then to recovery and how life has become a little different. Reading this book will help others embarking on this challenging and often exceptionally painful and even terrifying path—removing the mystery of "what to expect next" along with providing some tips to managing some of the very difficult things that go along with breast cancer treatment. However, I've never had breast cancer. My life has never been directly touched by anybody with any sort of cancer, which I suppose makes me some sort of unicorn, statistically. Yet, this book was wildly profound and important to me, because this book is not focused on surviving breast cancer as much as it is about living life through an empowering and hopeful spiritual approach. Cindy leads her readers through a series of Visualization Activities and Big Picture Processing questions that take you on a guided tour through a mode of spiritual and mindset empowerment that can be applied no matter what adversity you're facing in your life—breast cancer or literally anything else.

Cindy's writing on spirituality and lessons on using it to embrace all adversity with a spirit of empowerment and hope, speaks in a universal voice—told in such a way that would be embraced by most believers of Christianity, Islam, Hindi, Buddhism, Judaism, Unitarianism… nearly any belief system I can recall. This is a special gift, and one that I am deeply appreciative to have experienced through my immersion in The Pink Mountain. Through this work, my own perspective on leveraging my spirituality to approach all adversity through a sense of empowerment and hope has been awakened, and I hope the same experience is had by many others who have an opportunity to read this book. I encourage you, fellow readers, to actively take part in all of the activities that The Pink Mountain offers through your personal journey. While I have not yet had my life touched by breast cancer, I'm grateful that this resource is available for those who are battling through this journey and for their loved ones who would also benefit from this knowledge and mindset strategies. Here's to life—a temporary but brilliant adventure!

INTRODUCTION

As a woman going through breast cancer, I believe, the most powerful thing you can control is your perspective. In times like this, your strength and resiliency are tested to the max, and I truly believe that we each discover that we are much stronger than we think we are. When you're diagnosed with breast cancer, make no mistake, you have been victimized by breast cancer. The interesting thing is that even though that's true, you don't have to be a victim. You have the power to be a warrior and thrive through the journey in front of you. Choosing to thrive doesn't mean everything is sunshine and roses; it means that you don't have to sit in fear and feel powerless—you get to tap into an internal power that you never knew you had.

To me, being a warrior isn't about displays of brute force, a violent trope like we see in movies. Being a warrior is about choosing a mindset that empowers you to look fear in the eye, rise up, and be the best you can be, regardless of the situation. Every moment of everyday, you have the ability to choose your thoughts, your words, and your actions—these add up, creating the results in your life. You can't change the events happening in your life, but you can choose how you view, interpret and act upon them, thus impacting the results you get. In other words, while you can't change your breast cancer diagnosis, you can control how you respond to it and your experiences as you live through it.

Facing breast cancer is a hard journey that is filled with many unknowns, and it can feel like an impossible climb—steep and treacherous at times—which I call "The Pink Mountain". As a woman who has made it to the top of my Pink Mountain, I am here to tell you that if you are prepared mentally and emotionally, you will feel the power of your Spirit guiding you throughout your journey, regardless of where your finish point ends on the mountain. This book includes the strategies that I have used for myself and have guided many other women through to experience a more empowered and peaceful journey during an often terrifying and painful ascent.

In this book, you will be introduced to an awareness strategy that, when applied, will help you shift your perspective and allow you the opportunity to choose how you want to respond to the chaos and tumultuous landscape of the Pink Mountain. Like with any challenging climb, your ability to succeed is dependent upon your pre-climb preparation. When you are prepared, you can apply what you've learned to keep moving ahead in the right direction regardless of the rough terrain. This book provides you with a step-by-step process that you can use as your guide.

About Me

Supporting women going through breast cancer is what I do. Inspiring them to shift their perspective and see that they are stronger than they ever thought possible is who I am. My journey to the top of the Pink Mountain re-defined who I am and my purpose in life, and this book is literally my life's work—it's how I kept alive, sane, and empowered through something that truly seemed impossible at times.

My Diagnosis Story: It was July 2015, and I was cleaning up my desk. As I was sorting the mass of papers piled up, I came across my requisition for my yearly mammogram. I usually do this in February, but oops! I totally forgot about it! I phoned the imaging centre and scheduled myself for the next available appointment, which turned out to be August 12, my 45th Birthday. Yay! Nothing like getting your boobs pancaked on your birthday.

As I was heading out the door to go to my appointment, I realized that I had the time wrong. My appointment was actually an hour later than I was thinking it was. The schedule for the day was looking impossible, balancing work, this appointment, I needed to meet and work with my manager that morning, too. I couldn't do both, so I rescheduled my mammogram. It was no big deal, and a week later would be just fine.

Then, a week later finally arrived on a Wednesday, when I got my boobs squeeze done. The next day, Thursday, while I was at work doing a display build in one of the grocery stores, I received a call from my partner, Cheryl, who said that the imaging centre called, and I needed to call them back. Like every woman who gets a call back from imaging, I got a little nervous, thinking: hmmm WTF; that can't be good! Then, I gently reminded myself that over the years whenever I had a call back it was because they wanted better images. So, I called the appointment desk and scheduled myself for the next day. Then I started thinking more, still nervous, and since the next day was Friday and I'd have a whole weekend to panic about the new results, I called them back again and was able to get in later that same day — Thursday.

Thursday afternoon came, and as I was waiting for the imaging tech to come and get me, I was thinking how glad I was that I was able to get in now instead of Friday. I was still feeling a little anxious, but I knew that I would have answers sooner than later, and then I could put my brain to rest. Eventually, the tech came and got me, did more images on my left breast, and when I said thank you, have a good day, I was told that I couldn't leave yet—they were "squeezing me into" ultra sound.

I was the only one in the waiting room as my "squeeze in" was going to happen sometime over the lunch break. I was doing everything in my power to calm my catastrophic monkey mind from driving me to full-on panic. I went from *OMG I can't believe this is happening to me,* to, *it could be anything—it's probably nothing.* I tried calling my partner, Cheryl, but she didn't answer her phone, because she was in a chiropractor appointment. So then I thought I would call my friend, Susan, who answered right away, because she was waiting in a long line at the bank on a Thursday afternoon, so she had plenty of time to talk. When I told her where I was and what I was waiting for, there was a moment of dead silence. Her brain was racing to where my brain already was.

I remember telling her, "My 'Spidey Sense' is tingling. I have a very, very bad feeling about this."

As any good friend does, Susan did her best to run through a list of things it could be other than the C-word. While Susan was talking, I felt a shiver run through me, and I knew at a deep, intuitive level that it was cancer. As this realization was sinking in, I sipped in a deep breath and decided right then and there to stand tall and stare fear in the eye. I could not control whether or not I had cancer; the only thing I could control was how I chose to respond to it. I would not let fear rule me! I felt a sense of calm, like a warm blanket wrapped over me, and I knew that no matter the outcome of these tests, I would be okay.

Susan sensed a shift in my voice as we continued talking, and that shift told her that she could hang up, and I would be able to face whatever happened next. I got off the phone, and moments later, women started coming into the waiting room, ready to be called into whatever tests they were getting. When I looked at these women, I could see by their faces who was here for a routine test, who were having their first mammogram, and who were here for something… more. The lady who was reading the posters with very wide eyes, was clearly there for what must be her first mammogram, so I engaged her in conversation and helped settle any of her concerns. Talking to her also kept me in a calm frame of mind. As I panned the room to see who else might need some reassurance, I was called into the ultrasound room My "Spidey Sense" pinged again when it was a doctor instead of a tech doing the ultrasound.

I get why imaging doctors and techs won't tell you what they see, but that doesn't make it any less annoying. They think they talk in code, but it's not hard to crack their secret language and read between the lines. By the time I was done with the ultrasound, I knew that I had breast cancer. It was becoming evident to me in how the doctor was taking his time and saying we need to get clear images. Then, when he said, "While you are here let's ultrasound your lymph nodes because they will want to see that," my skin tingled. As he was finishing up, he told me that I would be getting called for a biopsy sometime next week. I was still trying to hold on to hope, and I told myself they will want to biopsy anything that looks suspect, and that it could be a cyst. It was when he left the room and a second later came back, put his hand on my shoulder and said, "I wish you the best of luck with everything," that I knew I would be facing the hardest climb of my life.

I left the imaging centre and went back to work. I had another display build to do across town, and life goes on. I remember feeling quite numb and very unsure about how I was feeling. One minute I would be scared thinking *OMG, this can't be happening to me.* Then the next thinking, *it's ok, you've got this.* Like hiking a mountain, just take one step at a time.

I went into the store to do the display build and carried on with my day as if that little episode didn't even happen. I did my best to ignore my monkey mind that wanted to bounce around thoughts of catastrophe and fear. This translated into unbridled nervous energy—I was wired! I didn't want to say anything to anyone about what was up, mostly because nothing had been confirmed and also, I wanted to take time to truly process my situation and understand the big picture before I dumped it onto others. I didn't want to create drama, which is what happens when people start shooting from the hip without any known target. Bullets fly everywhere, hitting everyone, causing chaos instead of a landing on a precise target.

With all of this nervous adrenaline pumping through me, I got through that build in record time! As I stood admiring my display, I was feeling proud that I successfully made it through the day with my brain in another dimension. Right then is when my phone rang—the call I was expecting but had momentarily forgotten, and it was Cheryl asking how things went at the imaging centre. I paused for a moment, and I wondered about the best way to answer Cheryl without causing her to get too upset, especially while she was home alone. I wanted to be upfront and direct but not create premature panic. I replied with, "Well, they are scheduling me for a biopsy sometime next week." It took Cheryl a few seconds to process what I said. I assured her that I was okay and that we would take one step at a time and we would figure things out. I know that in the time from when I hung up to when I got home, Cheryl would have gone through the ringer with her feelings. I had been processing things for the last six hours; Cheryl needed her chance.

By the time I got home, Cheryl was calm, and we were able to have a conversation about what tests they did, what the doctor said, and that we would not get too far ahead of ourselves until we knew more. Funny thing, I gave myself a self-exam that night, and there it was, I could feel the round lump that set off the alarms in the imaging centre. In my heart, I knew I had breast cancer, and I knew that I needed to get my game face on.

The next morning, I got a call confirming a biopsy appointment for that next Wednesday. In the meantime, I did start doing research. I went to reputable sites and educated myself. I wanted to make sure I had an understanding of the process, and possible outcomes. I am a big picture person. I like to see all aspects and angles so I can prepare myself for whatever gets thrown at me. At this point in the game, I looked up "biopsy", "DCIS" (stage 0) and "Stage I breast cancer". By the time I had my biopsy that Wednesday, I felt that I had a clearer understanding of what they were looking for, and I felt confident with the procedure itself. For the record, confidence with the procedure didn't make it any less painful. I'm just saying!

Listening to what the doctor was saying as he performed the biopsy, I was able to read between lines, and I knew that this wasn't going to be DCIS. I was hoping it was, but from the research I did, and from what he was doing in the biopsy, all signs were leading to—at minimum—a Stage I diagnosis. I had seven days to wait before I would know if my intuition was right or wrong.

The waiting in between had a lot of "what if" conversations, both alone with myself and with Cheryl. What if I need a lumpectomy? What if I need a mastectomy? What if I need chemo? When will this happen? We just booked our trip to Mexico, so will we still be able to go? If we can't, will we be able to get our money back? What will happen with my job? What if I don't get coverage because insurance companies are mean and like to make claims challenging? When Cheryl and I would sit down to talk, her what ifs were pretty similar to mine. At that point, we were just keeping things between the two of us.

I also believe in the power of knowledge, and I wanted to be prepared for any news the doctor would be giving us. I found that the research I was doing was helping me understand the bigger picture as well as helping me form educated questions to ask the doctor. The key here really is to ensure what research you undertake is from reputable sources—medical journals, articles from oncologists, and other sources that have provable reputations in the medical community. Misinformation and mythology are wide-spread, and it's critical to understand the difference when you embark on the journey of learning about what you're ultimately facing: breast cancer. The bigger picture requires understanding and knowledge, but you do need to ensure your sources are good.

Just to clarify, when I talk about understanding the bigger picture, this is about me taking a 360-degree, birds eye view of the situation. I want to have all my angles covered and all of the possible outcomes examined so that I am not surprised at any point in the process. For example, I researched the differences between Stage I and Stage II breast cancer. I pictured what my life would look like with Stage I, and when I did that, I knew I would get through it fine. Then I pictured life with a Stage II diagnosis, and when I did that, I knew I would get through it. It would be a harder journey than Stage I, but I knew I would get through it. I glanced at Stage III information, but I noticed that the treatment would be similar to Stage II, so I chose not to overwhelm myself with additional information and statistics.

I continued to talk and share my research findings with Cheryl. I wanted her to understand where I was in my thoughts, and I also wanted to help ease her mind from too much worry. I found that the more we shared, the more we would be prepared for whatever diagnosis I received.

A week later, I got my diagnosis, and I indeed had Invasive Ductal Carcinoma. I had breast cancer. At that point, we didn't know what Stage it was. That would come to light once I sat with the surgeon and talked about next steps. Even with all of the prep I did beforehand, actually hearing the doctor say those words felt like a shot in the stomach. They say always bring someone to your appointments, and now I know why. It takes a few moments to process the news. It's like you zone out, and you lose your hearing. The doctor is talking, you're nodding your head, but you really didn't hear anything he said for the last 30 seconds. Next thing you know, you're leaving the doctor's office in shock—not really aware of much in the moment. So, bringing a person to your appointments is critical, because they can help document and remember what you were told. Also, depending on the news you receive and your reaction to it, the other person can help with any emotional support needed and, in some cases, provide actual functional skills such as being oriented to where you are and driving home. Frankly, you don't know what news you will get sitting in that room, so it is best to have someone with you for countless reasons.

I began recalling what I learned in my research, and I knew that to successfully climb that beast of a mountain I would need to be grounded mentally, physically, emotionally and spiritually. I felt confident that all of the education, training, personal development and spiritual practice that I cultivated over the years had prepared me for the journey ahead. Even though my path ahead was filled with unknowns, I had a strong faith and knowingness that I would make it through.

Thrive the Climb

Hi, I'm Cindy: It was halfway through my chemo treatment when Cheryl asked me if I was really "this ok" with everything, because I hadn't had one single breakdown. I thought about it for a moment, and I recognized that it was true. I never even uttered the words "why me" once.

My calm and accepting manner to my breast cancer journey doesn't make me a hero or a robot. What it does tell me is that I have a way of successfully applying the concepts I have learned throughout my life to help shift my perspective and tune into my Spirit to get through challenging situations. If what I do has helped me so much, I want to share that with other women going through this same journey so they too can Thrive the Climb.

I have been consciously working on, blending, and applying "my" understanding of eastern and western wisdom to create powerful results out of everyday situations since 2009. This practice helped me gain insight into how Ego and Spirit like to show up, act, and influence the results we get in our lives. In short:

Ego thrives on fear and anger.

Spirit thrives on love and peace.

These two "voices" like to whisper in your ear every moment of every day. Whether you suffer or flourish in your life, no matter the challenges you're facing, depends on your awareness of these two voices and which one you feed and give power to the most.

Consciously hearing and listening to your Soul's guiding words, and choosing the high road of Spirit, is challenging when life is going fairly well, let alone under extreme stress. With my breast cancer diagnosis, I was about to embark on a stressful journey that would test me at every step. I knew I would have an epic battle between my Ego and Spirit. Yet, I had faith that through my dedicated "spiritual" practice, I had developed my self-awareness skills enough to keep Ego and its fear tactics from taking total control and sabotaging me while I climbed up that Pink Mountain. I expected to have many up and down moments, in fact, you need both extremes in all aspects of life to get a clear understanding of who you are and where you came from (Ego and Spirit make sure of this). For example, you would not know what happy is without the emotion of sad.

Like a rollercoaster, you need to have many ups and downs to have a thrilling ride.

What I experienced was that I was correct when I said it would be an epic battle between Ego and Spirit. I learned a great deal about myself because Ego showed up ready to play and take control of my thoughts, words and actions with its tricks and tactics, but at each turn, my Spirit was ready to fight back. Through every leg of the climb, I was challenged physically, emotionally, mentally and spiritually. As exhausted as I was, I felt blessed that my dedicated spiritual and self-awareness practice helped keep my connection to Spirit strong and shining bright throughout my climb.

I truly feel that it is my ability to shift my perspective at key moments that allows me to choose the mindset that best serves and supports me in those moments in time that would otherwise seem impossible. Teaching you this process so you can thrive through your breast cancer journey has brought me to write this book and develop programs to serve and support you.

About Reading "The Pink Mountain"

This book has been broken down into two parts to help you prepare and successfully scale up the Pink Mountain and reach the summit, whether that be triumphantly completing your cancer treatment, or graciously loving yourself for fighting hard to find and understand your true purpose.

You will notice that parts of the book are written in italics, and these are my personal stories that I wanted to differentiate from the rest of the content as living parallels to the experiences I had that may be similar to or very different from your own. Whether similar or different, I hope that they will give you a view into my thought processes, and how I came to the realizations that I did through this journey. Also, you will see excerpts from my journal, shown in handwritten font, and these journal entries provide you with a spotlight into my inner-thoughts as I climbed my own Pink Mountain.

Part One of this book is: "Pre-Climb Prep"

You will be introduced to what I call the Soul Games, and where you will also be gaining an understanding of your belief system. Soul Games is a strategical overview and layout of your current mindset, where it comes from, and the direct relationship it has to the results you are getting in your life, both past and present. This framing will help you get a solid idea on the workings of your belief system, which is the driver behind every thought, word and action you have.

From there I will be sharing a short story that I created, that will help paint a mental picture of each element of your belief system, how they mesh together and become that driver that creates your mindset.

Once you have a clear vision of who you are and what makes you tick, you will be shown awareness strategies, that when consciously used, will have a positive impact on all events in your life both past and present.

The final steps of pre-climb prep include a last-minute mindset check to reassess your current mental attitude, allowing you the opportunity to make any necessary adjustments if needed. You will also be shown and offered some equipment and resources that will help you find, lock in, and maintain your warrior mindset along the way.

Part Two of this book: "The Climb"

When I heard the words, "You have Invasive Ductal Carcinoma," I immediately pictured my journey to beating breast cancer as a climb up a big, daunting, massive mountain. This analogy made sense to me because I have hiked and climbed plenty of mountains over the years, and I know that even though getting to the top can be a challenge physically and mentally, the feeling of freedom for accomplishing such a feat empowers my Soul. The feeling of standing on what feels like the pinnacle of the world and looking down at the challenging terrain I just got through is indescribable. I measure it in terms of what it was like back to the start of the climb, where hours earlier I stood staring up at the peak of what seemed like an insurmountable quest, and now being at the top is a feeling of pure exhilaration in achievement. Literally, just putting one foot in front of the other, with grit and determination, got me to the top of the mountain. The impossible was possible!

With the challenges of your journey being unknown, taking it one step at a time will get you up the mountain. Throughout your cancer journey, you will make sure you have knowledge of the terrain by learning and educating yourself on all possible angles so you can adapt to any sudden changes. If you understand the hazards, you can do a better job at staying on track. If you choose to listen to your heart and soul, and maintain a strong climbing mind and body, you will grow throughout your journey. You will not just survive, you will thrive!

You will feel the empowerment of standing on top of this beast of a mountain, knowing that you just stretched yourself in ways you didn't even know were possible. In your most trying moments you persevered, kept your feet moving, and in the end, learned a lot about yourself in every sense of your being. To help you stay aware of your Soul Games and to stay on track throughout your climb, you will be answering a series of questions at the start of each chapter in this part of the book, which I call Big Picture Processing (BPP). This is a grounding method to condense the knowledge you learned in the Pre-Climb, so you can quickly and effectively check in and process yourself to determine which mindset you want showing up for you.

As you work your way through each leg of the climb, you will learn a lot about yourself. If you remain open and apply what you have learned in your pre-climb prep, you will notice a strength coming from within that will lovingly guide and push you through your hardest times.

PART 1:
Pre-Climb Prep

CHAPTER 1:

Life

You are going to notice that I talk a lot about "time/space events", "dualities" and "understanding the big picture". I am going to get a little metaphysical and next-level for a second, as I would like to share my thoughts and beliefs around the "bigger picture" when talking about life. Being open and willing to explore these concepts will help you build a solid foundation to get all you can out of the Pre-climb prep.

As long as I can remember, when it came to learning complex subjects, if I broke down the key concepts into examples or analogies that resonated in "my language," I would have greater success in understanding and enjoying the subject being presented. Over the years of learning and growing, I have honed my craft of creating analogies that help crush the complexity of this subject matter for myself and others.

When I read self-realization or personal development books, I find I have to re-read the passages several times. I know the concepts the author is sharing are essential, and they need to not only be understood, but applied. For me, I find that when I put the essence of the message into analogies that "my" brain can understand, I instantly get that A-ha moment and feel a vibrating energy ripple through my body. Once this shift happens, my mind, body and spirit align, and I know that not only do I understand the author's message, but I am now conscious enough to apply it if I so choose.

For instance, women often seek guidance to navigate their lives with greater success, but we can get lost in the "technical language and psychology" of personal development. They also know it takes time and great focus to read, decipher and learn this intricate subject. I know first-hand of the committed effort it takes to walk though those muddy waters, and spend time filtering it, until it becomes clear and life-sustaining. I am able to help women shift their perspective and see their challenges in a new light, because I take and share life altering wisdom and experiences that I have cultivated over years of reading and study, and I present it in a way that helps paint a clear picture for them to connect with, and feel their a-ha moment rapidly.

Throughout this book I will be sharing complex, self-realization concepts, in words that are relatable and actionable—like a conduit from an energy source to the thing that needs power. Through personal examples and colorful analogies, I hope to inspire you to view life as a great adventure, full of learning opportunities that enrich your life along the way. May this book be a lustrous stepping stone, that not only gets you up the Pink Mountain but also leads you on a path of continued self-discovery to your inner strength and power.

Let's explore "experience" for a moment. To me heaven is a word to describe the "Absolute". The Absolute is a dimension in time and space that offers your Soul the experience of oneness and connection with your higher power. That higher power is known by many names, and God is one of them. In the Absolute, you are pure love and light. This isn't your experience on Earth, of course, because if you are always pure love and light, you will never understand the true experience of it without its antithesis. You must have an experience to compare it against for you to understand, value, and nurture these values. Like any being, the desire to feel, understand and know who you are and where you fit into the bigger picture becomes overwhelming. The Supreme Being, the creator it is, created the "Relative" world that you call earth.

In contrast, this Relative world is intelligently designed so that you can experientially know who you are in relation to everyone and everything else. Every relationship you have made, whether it's a smile to someone on the street or conversations with your closest friend--even your interactions with the environment and all the species in it—gives you the opportunity to understand and know who you are. There are two parts of this intelligent design that you will examine throughout this book: 1) Time/space events and 2) Dualities.

Think of time/space in terms of it being a puzzle—a real puzzle. So, imagine yourself going into a hobby store to buy a jigsaw puzzle. As you scan the shelf, you see an image that grabs your attention. You are attracted to everything about it: the colors, the texture and the beautiful picture that speaks to your Soul. Walking out of the store, you are thrilled with your purchase and can't wait to get home to start creating the image that was promised on the cover of the box.

As you know, there is no right or wrong way to put a puzzle together; however, once you've put a few together, you have figured out a system that seems to work for you. You've likely based this system on trial and error as well as some guidance from other puzzle goers. Plus, there are a few steps that seem universal, right? The first thing you do when you open the box is spread out the puzzle pieces face side up so that even though you don't know what the little images are that are looking at you right away, you know with time and patience, eventually these seemingly random bits will fit together, and you will complete the puzzle and the beautiful picture will come together.

You keep the cover near-by in case you need to refer back to it for guidance, but for the most part you are lovingly scanning and going from piece to piece, intuitively selecting the right one at the right time to complete whatever section of the puzzle you are working on. Every now and then you pick up a piece that you think is the right one and you feverishly try to make it fit. Eventually you come to your senses and put it aside, then keep looking. The right piece is usually the one you overlooked ten times before actually picking it up, or it's one you already tried, but it didn't seem to fit then, but for whatever reason it magically worked this time.

Eventually, you start to see the different parts of the puzzle images come into focus. You are starting to get a glimpse of the bigger picture. You don't even find it necessary to look at the box cover anymore, it's like you and the puzzle are one. As the puzzle image is emerging and the pieces are getting fewer, you are getting excited to finish. It's been a long, fun, frustrating and exciting process. There were many times you were tired of it all and wanted to give up, but you stuck with it. Now, as you are down to the final piece, you feel a sense of pride and accomplishment for your efforts. You step back and look at your hard work and smile. You did it! You created the beautiful image as promised on the cover of the box.

Sometimes you tear apart the puzzle right away, or if the puzzle has been extra hard, you decide to keep it up for the day to admire it and enjoy the feeling of achievement. This puzzle is one to keep up for the day!

By the next morning, walking past the puzzle you smile at it, and then you lovingly tear it apart. You know that you are ready to tear it down, and you need to make room for the experience of the next puzzle. Like the beautiful picture on the box and the pieces of the jigsaw puzzle, your time/space events are the experiences your Soul needs to have so it can experience the beauty of who it is. Time/space events are countless pieces of the big picture that your Soul created and spread out over time and space. Throughout your life you will have ample opportunity to pick up the pieces and create the beautiful picture your Soul desires. The more you become aware of the pieces you are holding, the more efficient you will be at connecting everything together.

The other essential ingredient of life in this Relative world is dualities. Simply put, dualities are opposites. For example, you can't understand what hot is without having the experience of its opposite: cold. You can't understand what happiness is without the experience of sadness. You can't understand what the feeling of healthy is without the experience of illness. You can't experience Love without Fear, Spirit without Ego and Warrior without Victim. So, as much as you dislike the negative experiences you have faced, it is wise to look at them as a blessing. For without them, you would have nothing to compare yourself to and would struggle to interpret and put together the pieces of the bigger picture that your Soul is here to experience.

I will be using personal stories and analogies throughout this book to help demonstrate how understanding your bigger picture will enable you to look at life from a higher perspective. As you begin to connect the dots of your time/space events and dualities, you will see the beauty and perfection unfold. You will witness the evolution of your Soul through You!

CHAPTER 2:

The Bigger Picture

Why in the world would your Soul actually choose to have cancer as part of its experience, or any traumatic, life altering event for that matter? Really, who would choose that? Here is the thing—only your Soul knows what the picture on the cover of the box looks like, and your time/space events fit its plan perfectly. Metaphorically speaking, your job is to become aware of the images on the puzzle pieces by becoming consciously aware of your time/space events. That way you can begin to put the pieces together and see your Soul's purpose—Its bigger picture.

Being consciously aware means being aware of the Soul Games and choosing the mindset you apply to your time/space events. Essentially, you only have two choices. If you are coming from a Warrior Mindset, you have embraced the path of your Spirit. You will lovingly care about your Soul's puzzle pieces and work at completing the bigger picture. If you are coming from a Victim Mindset, you are walking the path of your Ego. You will either haphazardly pick up and try to jam incorrect puzzle pieces together, or you will ignore the Soul's calling entirely, with Ego's fear-filled agenda. Either mindset will provide you with a result in life, but it is up to you to choose which path you take. The path to a beautiful creation or the path to a gloomy, doomsday existence is your choice. It will always be your choice. Understanding the Soul Games, your belief system and doing some awareness strategies will help you tap into your

Warrior Mindset so you can consciously choose to put the puzzle pieces together and enjoy the beauty that unfolds.

This chart gives an overview of the Soul Games as mentioned above. This gives you a map to your mindset. Keep this page bookmarked as it is also a reference for you to see and connect the different names and concepts I will be referring to throughout this book.

Soul Games

(Mindset Map)

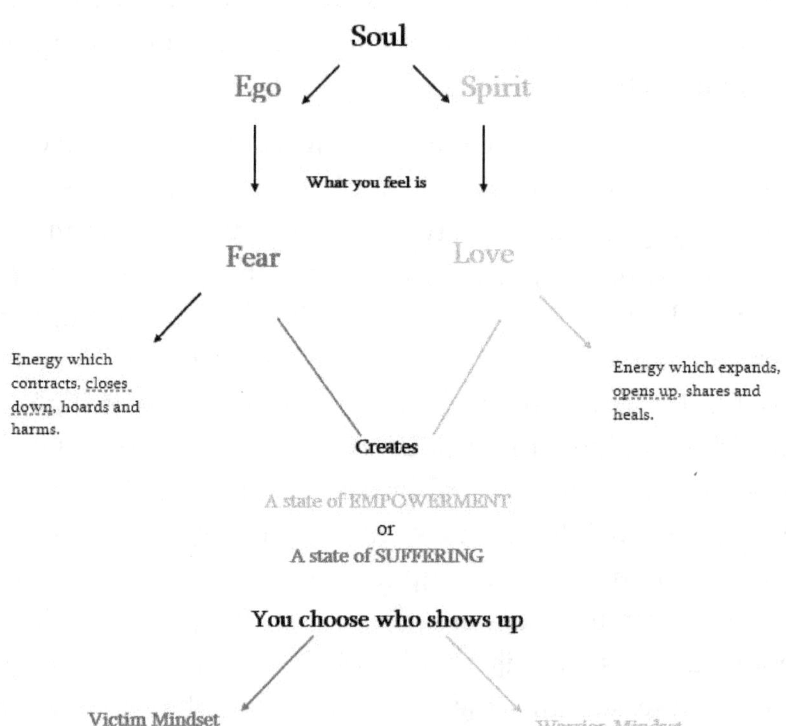

AUTHOR'S NOTE: Throughout this book, I will repeat concepts in many different ways. Repetition is the key to learning and mastering any skill. By the end of your climb with cancer and in life, you will have a greater understanding of your Soul's purpose and the beauty and perfection that lies within.

CHAPTER 3:

Cancer, Your Life, and the Soul Games

What is your diagnosis story? Did you journal your experience? No? Do it now. Visualize yourself back in all of those appointments, tests and picture yourself in the moment you got your diagnosis and journal about it. BE AS DETAILED AS YOU CAN and take as much time as you need. Once you finish journaling, read through your experience and create a list of the words that describe how you felt then and also how you are currently feeling—emotionally, physically, and spiritually feeling. Please keep the list handy as we will be referring back to it later in the book.

Just to be clear, there is no right or wrong way to feel. Feelings are the language of the Soul. They are expressed as thoughts and words, and when you pay attention, you have the opportunity to gain an understanding of your location in the Soul Games, and then you can decide if it's where you want to be. If you miss that first level of opportunity, you do have a second level, which is, looking at the results you are getting in your life, which will quickly determine if your feelings are indeed supporting you or not. To clarify—check in with your feelings and identify exactly what they are, without judging them. Write it down in a journal to really explore them. If what you are feeling isn't serving your goal, you have an opportunity to shift your feelings for a different result.

Think about this: when you heard the words, "you have breast cancer," how did you feel? How shocked were you? Did you feel yourself rise up, and while you knew you were going to be facing the hardest climb of your life, did you have a sense of calm in knowing that all you could do is take one step at a time and you would deal with things as they came? Or did you feel out-of-control, panic and fear, that your life just took a terrible turn, and you were now just a passenger, powerless, on a ride to hell? Generally, people tend to feel only one way or the other, and both are valid.

Yet, the reactions are so very different. Why do some women react one way to their cancer diagnosis while others respond in another way? It is because your thoughts, words and actions are coming from either Love or Fear, which is shaped by your Spirit or Ego. Everything you have learned from these two entities has been preserved inside of you as your belief system. The feelings you get are your Soul's way of letting you know if you are being divinely guided by Spirit or pulled around by Ego. Your feelings are expressed by the words you use both internally (what you say to yourself) and externally (what you verbally express). You are dialed into these frequencies like stations on a radio. So how do you know who's whisper you are tuned into?

The only way to know the answers to these questions is by examining the results you are getting in your life. Remember, there is no such thing as a wrong or right result in your life; it all comes down to what is working or not working for you. For example, there are some areas of your life where things are running smoothly, and you are happy and pleased as punch. Chances are, in these areas, you are showing up with a warrior mindset. Yet, in other parts of your life, you just can't seem to get it together or catch a break. It seems like things are always happening to you, and you are miserable. Most likely, in these parts, you are showing up with a victim mindset. You begin to search for ways to cheer yourself up, and quite often this usually involves an external fix, such as drugs, alcohol or excessive consumerism. The only sustainable way to change your results is to become aware of how you are showing up in the game of life, particularly in areas that plague you with feelings of fear or powerlessness. You need to see and understand why these events keep coming up, so you can choose to respond differently. To do that, you need to be aware of the "chatter" you hear being whispered in your mind and the belief system attached to those voices.

In psychology, the terms Ego, Id, Super Ego, Conscious, Subconscious and Superconscious are used to describe the chatter of your mental awareness. There are a lot of levels and complexities to each one of these areas, but to keep things easy to understand, and forward moving, you will focus on Ego mostly right now. In your mind, picture Ego as a character sitting on your left shoulder, and she looks and sounds just like you. You call this dark, sly character Shade. Shade is one of the voices whispering in your ear, and you have been hanging out together since you came into this world. You have seen and done a lot over the years and have developed such a comfortable relationship that you even subconsciously let this little spitfire make most of your decisions. Yes, really! Well, of course you did—how much easier could it be for you to just show up and go along with whatever situation you find yourself in, letting fear and impulse guide you? Sometimes these situations work out for you, of course, but more times than not, you find yourself frustrated by the resulting shenanigans. Instead of questioning the antics of the sly character pulling you around, you instead choose to listen to the excuses and stories that Shade comes up with, and then lash out at the people around you, blaming them for your predicaments. Over time, these stories build up, and soon you are compulsively a victim to life, being led around subconsciously by Shade, watching precious time on earth go by while sitting on the sidelines, taking punches and getting angry but not making much progress.

Now, while Shade is causing you some troubles and issues in life, it is important to realize that having an Ego is not evil or even counter-productive. In fact, without Shade you wouldn't be able to fully experience who you are. The world has been intelligently designed for you to experientially learn who you are in relation to it. You don't know what something is until you experience its opposite. Remember the concept of dualities that we talked about earlier: you wouldn't know hot without cold, up without down, night without day, here without there, space without earth, love without hate, big without little, black without white, happy without sad, peace without war, light without dark, etc. This dichotomy holds true for your mind as well. Without Ego, we would not know our Spirit. You need the antithesis of a thing to fully experience it.

Again, keeping things simple, picture your Spirit as a warrior sitting on your right shoulder. Think of it as another character that plays a part in your life, one that looks and sounds just like you. You call this enlightened and powerful essence Blaze. You and Blaze have also been hanging out since you came into existence. Together, you have done and seen amazing things over the years and have a comfortable relationship. Unlike Shade, Blaze doesn't make decisions for you, but instead helps guide you to become aware of how you are showing up at the events in your life. This awareness is important because every moment of every day is loaded with opportunities for you to experience who You Are by becoming aware of the drama and shenanigans that Shade likes to create and realizing there is an opposite. Every event in your life is laced with lessons and outcomes designed specifically for your Soul to learn, grow and create and with the help of Blaze, you will manifest an abundant life filled with happiness and love.

Once you start to understand and truly "get" the importance of the dualities concept and see how the essence of everything (your relationships and time/space events) is designed for you to experientially learn who you are, you come from a place of power instead of fear. That is the essence of empowerment, so when you find yourself slipping, feeling powerless, fearful, and out-of-control, Spirit is calling for you to return to your inner-strength.

Shade is very sly and plays deceptive mind games with you in an attempt to control you and keep you in a small comfort zone—whether healthy or not, familiarity is always comforting. The smaller the playground, the better your left shouldered friend can keep your thoughts and experiences contained, which often leads to feelings of fear, anger, anxiety and depression. This isn't wrong, but if you are wanting to break out of your bubble and experience life to the fullest, then it's important to be aware of the Ego tactics that Shade uses. To do that you need to expand your playground and become BEST friends with Blaze.

So how do you do that? How do you just expand your playground? You need to become consciously aware of your thoughts, words, and actions, along with the belief system that shaped them.

Spirit is Love and gives rise to your thoughts that contain the highest joy, truth, peace, compassion, blessings and harmony.

• Words from Spirit contain energy that expands, opens up, shares and heals.

• Action from Spirit comes from a Warrior Mindset, creating results that support you in life and through your journey.

Ego is Fear and gives rise to your thoughts that contain sadness, lies, turmoil, torment, unforgiveness and drama.

• Words from Ego contain energy that contracts, closes down, hoards and harms.

• Action from Ego comes from a Victim Mindset, creating results that limit you in life and often leaves you stuck, preventing you from progressing on your journey.

Looking at your diagnosis story and your list of feelings, you can now see if you are tuned into Shade or Blaze. If you don't like what you are feeling or the results you are getting, you have the power to change who you are dialed into. Becoming aware of where you are now is important, because you can't successfully read a map and reach your destination without knowing your starting point.

CHAPTER 4:
Your Belief System, Your Starting Point

What is your belief system, and where did it come from?

Your belief system is your value system, which helps guide you through life. Its origin came from the opinions of everyone and everything you have experienced, beginning with infancy, progressing into your toddler years through to childhood, and then all the way through your formative years and beyond into your teens. Your beliefs are essentially the container that surrounds you framing your attitudes and behaviors. Your beliefs shape your thoughts, words, and actions that create the results in your life. In short, your belief system is the driver behind your thoughts and feelings.

Below is a diagram depicting the framework of how your belief system works and why you get the results you are currently getting in your life. I call this your Belief System Cycle:

Belief System Cycle.

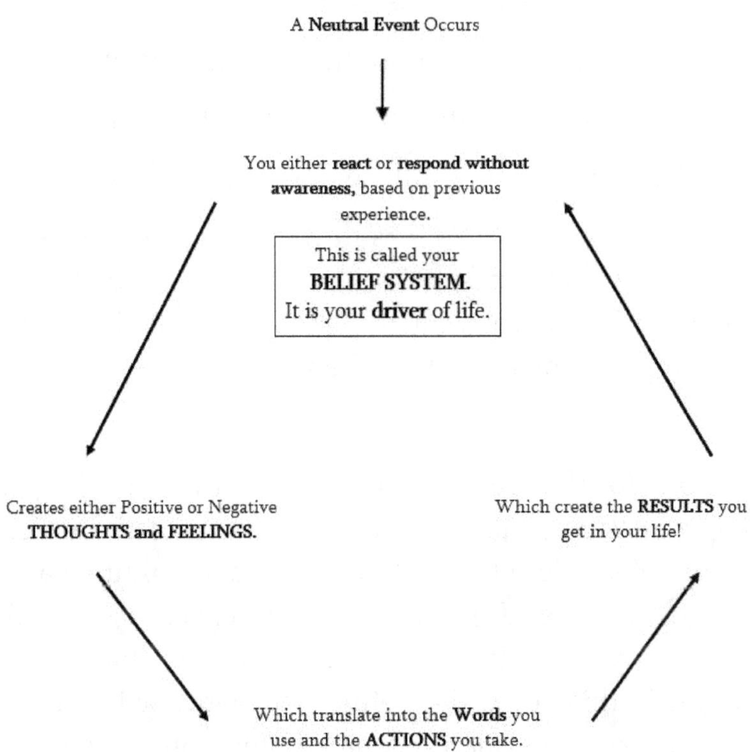

There are a series of steps involved here and understanding how they interact is important if you desire to make a shift in the results you're currently experiencing, and for future experiences.

Here is the step-by-step process that links everything together:

Step 1: A neutral event occurs (Your time/space event) →

Step 2: Your belief system kicks in →

Step 3: Which creates your thoughts and feelings →

Step 4: Which translate into your words and actions →

Step 5: Which create the results in your life →

Here is where the "cycle" kicks in… You will then respond or react without awareness to those results, and the cycle continues until you "consciously" choose differently, beginning with shifting your belief system (Step 2).

Definitions for this book—it's important that we all agree on what specific terms mean for the purposes of communicating effectively. You might think of these terms differently based on your life experiences thus far, which is fine, because just like in dictionaries you'll find that many words have several meanings. In this book, the definitions below will help us all keep these terms in a shared context. This is important so that we're all communicating in the same sphere of thought as we move forward:

1. Neutral event: Is a time/space event created just for you, so you can experientially know who you are in relationship to this world during this lifetime. While there may be more than one person involved in your neutral event, each individual will experience it differently, because each person's Soul has its own journey and lessons to learn from each event.

The term neutral event is just that, it's neutral. You will either react (negatively) or respond (positively) to the event based on your belief system, which determines your experience and outcome. You bring the energy to the neutral event!

2. Belief System: Is your personal container of knowledge. This container encompasses your entire working system of life that you began developing since your birth on earth. Your experience of life has created your values, as well as how you see and interpret the world.

This is the context you have developed and architected over your lifetime, and it either supports or limits you in achieving your Soul's purpose.

This complex system serves as the life support, like the roots of a tree, that feed your thoughts and feelings. Major life-decisions often are made for you based on what is feeding this system without you even being aware of it. Sometimes, this unconscious behavior works out for you, but most of the time you are just being pulled around and not even aware of how you are showing up in life. You're living passively versus intentionally until you develop a deeper awareness, which this book is designed to open for you.

3. Thoughts and Feelings: Your thoughts and feelings create either positive or negative energy. This energy sets into motion a cascade of intricacies, which will massively affect your life experiences and results that will either support you or limit you.

4. Words and Actions: Words happen internally or externally, and they add power to and eventually manifest your thoughts and feelings. Actions bring your thoughts, feelings and words to life, immediately, which ultimately leads to the results you are getting in your life.

5. Results: The results you get in life are the sum total of your current belief system manifested. If you do not like the results you are getting in your life, it's time to start paying attention to how you are showing up, and that means to take inventory of how your Spirit is aligned or not aligned with your thoughts, feelings, and actions.

So, now that our terminology is set, let's get into a little "real talk": What does understanding your belief system have to do with breast cancer? Everything! You can't change your cancer diagnosis, but you can change your attitude about it. You get to choose if you want to show up as a victim (Shade) or a warrior (Blaze), and to do this, you first need to become aware of your current belief system and determine if it is supporting or limiting you.

The moment you become aware of your thoughts and feelings is the moment you give yourself the option to choose your mindset. I am going to share an experience I had in this last year that really demonstrates the power of this awareness.

My Story: Adventures in Cozumel

I have always been somewhat adventurous and while we were in the Mexican Rivera this past January (2018) we decided to take the ferry across to Cozumel to enjoy some snorkeling. Now, I am not the strongest swimmer by any means. In fact, if you were to ask my partner Cheryl, she would tell you I swim like a rock. However, there is something truly mesmerizing about the crystal clear, azure waters, filled with colorful fish, that begs for the weakest of swimmers to throw on some fins, slap on a mask and become one with the ocean. Even though I lack swimming skills, I felt confident in the rest of my athleticism to join in on the quest to see the underwater universe that the island of Cozumel had to offer.

We were at one of the reef's and the snorkeling area was roped off and about the size of a football field. Excitedly we entered the water and began our adventure. We were out for about 40 minutes and decided to come back in for a rest. As we sat in our loungers, we decided that the next snorkel would be on the opposite side of the grid that we just experienced. After 30 minutes we geared up again and explored the reef and beyond.

After about 40 minutes I signaled to Cheryl that we should start heading back. For some reason it felt harder. To avoid running into the reef I started moving outwards at a 10 degree angle, so the current would land me in front of the entry dock. After what seemed like forever, I lifted my head up to see where I was. I couldn't believe it I was still a long way away from the dock. All that effort and kicking and I didn't get far at all. I figured the current was changing, so I just kept moving. Again, when I looked up, I was way off my target. I knew I was running out of steam so I gave all I could to get me back to safety. After what felt like forever, I lifted my head to check my progress.

WTF! How could the dock still be way over there?! I had gotten so far off course that I was now in the opposite side of the football field.

Stunned at how I could have gotten so off course, I tore off my mask and snorkel to get a better look. I couldn't believe what I was seeing.

The whole time I was lifting my head, I was actually looking at the wrong dock. I overshot my dock by a huge margin! That was when I realized I was in a world of trouble. I was in no man's land! I had no gas left in my tank, I completely exhausted myself swimming and by taking my mask off I took off the only thing that was helping me stay somewhat buoyant. I couldn't get my mask back on, and I started to panic. Fear ripped through me like lightening. OMG, this is it! This is how it's going to end! I am going to drown on my vacation in Mexico.

I couldn't even yell for help. I felt a heavy pressure starting to surround and compress my chest. My legs were working hard to keep my head up. The only thing I could do was gasp. Every movie I have seen with people drowning flashed through my mind. I was going down; I was literally going to drown! I had fleeting thoughts about everything that I hadn't completed in my life. I can't die yet! I pictured my partner Cheryl and the pain that she would have to go through. I could not [bleeping] believe that this was how my life was going to end.

As terror continued ripping through the fibers of my body, I could feel my legs slow, and I started to sink. This was it; my life was ending. In the moment of silence that followed that thought, a voice lifted me up: "You didn't climb through breast cancer to die here and now! Fight! Fight hard! You have a story to tell. You have some work to do!"

A complete calmness washed over me. I slowed my breath down and started moving. I thought just keep moving! I didn't know if I was going to make it or not, but I had to try. As I got closer to shore, I heard Cheryl screaming my name. I gasped her name, and after hollering at me, in relief, she started to make her way out to me. That was when I felt myself touching ground. I was touching ground! I fought hard, and I am touching ground. I am still alive! I conquered my fear, rose to the challenge, and I fought with everything I had.

As I sat in the beach lounger, trying to make sense out of what I just experienced, I felt so many feelings and thought so many thoughts. In all of my personal and spiritual development, I know that when your time is up, it is up. You can't stop your Soul from moving on.

When your time is done here on earth, it is done. That voice I heard in that moment of silence was my Soul fighting to continue existing as the Spirit Cindy. It was not ready to move on. Apparently, I still have some learning, growing and creating to do. It was not my time!

The Parallel

Do you see the similarities? When you were diagnosed, did you feel like you were drowning and gasping for breath? That parallel was not lost on me, either…

Even though you were standing on land when you got your diagnosis, you were fighting to breathe. You were scared and felt like you were alone, in the middle of "no man's land" with nothing to hang on to. You may or may not have had a physical person by your side, but trapped in that moment, you are undeniably alone, regardless. Your life flashed before your eyes, and you felt like your life was ending. Still, amid the confusion, you managed to regain your senses and bring yourself back to reality. Except now, reality is full of fear. Fear of the unknown. Fear that in any moment you are going to be told the news that will confirm your fears and completely rock your world for the worse. You literally can't move on with your life, because you are paralyzed by fear.

By the way, please don't judge yourself. All of this is normal in the moment. The point is to try not to get stuck there!

Being run by fear is just one way of thinking. That mindset is for real, but it isn't the only mindset. Every moment of everyday you consciously or unconsciously choose how you want to show up in life. You can either be pulled around in fear by your Ego and live life from a Victim mindset. Or, you can be guided from love by your Spirit, and live life from a Warrior Mindset. I want to be clear, there is nothing wrong with feeling the fear, but if it is having a negative impact on your life, that is your cue that you need to shift your mindset. In my story above from Mexico, had I stayed in fear and not shifted my mindset, I would have died and wrecked a perfectly good vacation!

If I had let Ego have its way, I would have had a premature death. I feel blessed that I was able to tune into the voice of my Spirit and fight my way back. As I sat looking over the ocean, I recognized that I got through my breast cancer journey the same way. I engaged my inner warrior and I fought my way back to shore. I made up my mind in the imaging centre that I wasn't going to go down in fear. If I was going to die from breast cancer, I wanted to do it knowing I embraced all of who I was, that I lived fully to my last breath, and be at peace knowing that my Soul was ready to move on.

We all have been victimized in life but that doesn't mean we have to choose a Victim Mindset. The ocean victimized me, but I didn't become a Victim. Breast cancer victimized me, but I didn't become a Victim. Can you feel the difference in that statement?

YOU have been victimized by breast cancer, but you DO NOT have to be a VICTIM.

The good news is you have the personal power to choose differently! You do not have to stay stuck with your current limiting beliefs. You have the opportunity to learn right here, right now, how to tap into your Warrior Mindset and not only scale this Pink Mountain, but also live your life from the voice of Spirit in all areas of your life moving forward.

CHAPTER 5:

How I Came to Be

Explaining the unexplainable, such as the essence of you as a human being, your indoctrination into this relative world, and how all of your early training has formed a foundation, just like the root system of a tree, which also allows you to grow branches, reaching out and expanding throughout all of your life. As natural a phenomenon as this is, it can also be exceptionally challenging when you want to take charge and live purposefully. That is why I created this short story called "How I Came to Be". As the reader, you will be inserting yourself into the story as a participant while also becoming the observer. This will allow you to immerse yourself into a 360-degree experience of who you are and how you came to be.

This story is designed to provide you with an understanding of where your belief system was birthed and how it has carried over, impacting your current mindset while creating the results in your life. You will also notice the connection between how learning to shift your perspective to becoming the observer in your own world gives you a new framework for becoming a Warrior in all areas of your life. As you become aware of your Belief System Cycle and the critical juncture into the Soul Games, this gives you the ultimate power to choose which mindset you want to show up with in life.

Short Story: How I Came to Be

Part 1: Visualization Activity—The Party

You are invited to a party, not just any party, this is THE party. Everyone is going to be there. It is the "who's who" event of the year!

I want you to picture yourself getting dressed and preparing yourself for a night out that you will never forget. I want you to notice how you feel as you are heading out the door and on your way to the party. En route, you begin to visualize what you are going to say to these "larger than life" people and how you are going to behave. You arrive, and as you are coming up the stairs and through the front doors, you find yourself over-the-top with excitement. You can't wait to see WHO is going to be at this party and how your life is going to change.

You enter into the room, and the first people you see are your parents. You think to yourself, *what are they doing at this party?* As your eyes start to circle the room, you see your grandparents, your brother and sisters, your school teachers, (even the ones you didn't like), your best friends, classmates, and even your worst enemies! You begin to ask yourself, *what kind of party is this?*

As you walk further into the room, you see the familiar face of your spouse, and just further past, you see the managers and owners of the different companies you've worked for, even the customers you had dealt with over the years. In one corner of the room, you hear music playing. As you draw closer, you realize that this is the exact music that you have listened to and enjoyed over the years. Music that you related to over different periods of your life. Some of those tunes got you through your darkest moments and some of them celebrated with you through your best moments. Turning to go deeper into the room, you walk past people you recognize from the grocery store, the coffee shop, gym and other places you regularly visit. You even notice people that look familiar, but you just can't quite place them.

You wander towards the refreshment table, and you see that it is lined with magazines. As you get closer, you notice that it is a collection of all the magazines and books you have read over the years. The advice in these publications helped you learn how to dress fashionably, how to win friends and how to meet and capture the perfect mate. They even helped to point out all of the things you did wrong in your life, providing a new, self-aware perspective for change.

Just then, you hear distracting voices coming from a different room. As you approach closer, you realize that these are voices of the celebrities and movie stars familiar to you. Finally, you think, Oh! *That's where the who's who of this party is hanging out!* Excitedly, you rush into the room, and instead of being met by the trend-setters and most influential people in the world, because the magazines said that they were, you are greeted by thousands of TV screens playing the movies and TV shows that you grew up watching over the years. Shows that taught you what life was about, entertained you and provided models for relationships and conflicts along with all of the other human interactions that seem so mysterious until you live them. Just when this party couldn't be any more bizarre, you notice a door with your name on it. This has struck your attention, and your curiosity is piqued. You move swiftly towards that door, but along the way, you take another look at the people in the room.

As you do this, you suddenly find yourself filled with different emotions as you remember the moments you shared with these people. Some people in the room you feel a true love for, and others you don't want anything to do with. Again, you are trying to figure out why all of these people are at this party.

You arrive at the door with your name on it. As you put your hand on the knob, you take one last glance over your shoulder and notice that the room has magically transformed into a long corridor of doors. Everyone at the party has their own door, with their name on it, and they too are heading into their own rooms!

Opening the door, you walk into a room that has wall-to-wall, old black and white movie reels playing. You examine them more closely, and you realize that everything in these films looks familiar, as though you were experiencing Deja vu. That's when you realize that these aren't just any movies—these are YOUR movies. They are clips from your life! All of the moments of your life are now playing before you. Your eyes grow wider as you begin to notice that all of the people from this strange party are in your clips!

As you watch the movie reels, a brilliant rainbow of emotions flow through you. You are reliving every moment and every event, with all of those people, as though it was happening for real, right now. The clips that are causing you the greatest agitation are the events where you felt angered, disappointment, criticized, laughed at, ridiculed, devastated, afraid. Suddenly, in a blink of an eye, the clips go from black and white to vivid color. The scenes pan back and you can now see yourself in the clips. You are watching the movies from a third person's perspective, as if you're just a member of an audience watching from a distance. You now have a bird's-eye-view of every event in your life!

From this angle, you begin to notice the details around you. The clues you never picked up on at the time of the actual event, such as the pain and anguish reflecting in the other person's eyes. That's when it hits you. You can now "see" the event from a "neutral" point of view. From this angle, you get an understanding of the other person's view, "if" you choose to look.

The devastating emotions that you felt from being in those crushing situations, suddenly start to fade as you realize that your version of the event was not necessarily the only version. From this perspective, you can actually see and feel what the other person was experiencing and why. By taking a step back, you are able to see that if you hadn't been so caught up in your own version, and took the time and effort to understand that everyone views the world differently, you could have learned something valuable from that person and event beyond just your own emotions, thoughts, fears, and needs!

You begin to ask yourself how could a neutral event trigger so much emotion? How is it that for all of these years, you thought your version of what transpired throughout your life was the only true and honest version of those events? What kind of party is this? Just then, you get a flash of insight and understanding: Everyone at the party is in their own room, seeing reels of their lives. If they have the strength and fortitude to get past their initial rainbow of emotions, they too will get to see their lives from a bird's-eye-view. They too, will get the opportunity to see that there are multiple sides to every story, and for every devastating event that we experience, there is a silver lining to all of our rainbows of emotion! Recognizing the importance of having a bird's-eye-view and the powerful lessons you can learn from them, you feel a strong desire to see everything through this lens at all times. As you glance back at the reels, you notice that the last reel playing is you in this very room, and the footage ends with you going through a door!

As you turn to the right, you see the door that the "you" in the movie reel went through. You open the door and step into the next room. You can't see anything in that room, but you feel a string hanging down. You pull the string, and light fills the room, and just as quickly as the light switches on, you are greeted by your reflection in a mirror. You slowly turn around the room and everywhere you look, your eyes are staring back at you. You realize that the whole room is made of mirrors. The mirrors not only hold your current image, but every image of you, from every moment through-out your life.

As you circle the room, some reflections you remember as being the happiest moments of your life, and they are staring back at you. In these images, you have a sparkle in your eyes while standing tall with confidence. You are radiating warmth and love. In the other reflections, which you recall as your saddest or most fearful moments, your eyes are pained, your body language is closed off, and the energy radiating from you feels cold and fearful. You lean in to take a closer look at the cold image staring back at you, and you realize that it isn't really you. At first glance, it looks like you, but there are slight differences in your eyes and body language. Just as you are asking yourself who this imposter is, your college psychology lectures pop into your mind. You also get flashes of information from the personal development books you'd read.

You know the answer. The imposter, in the reflections of the saddest moments of your life, is your Ego!

Ego is the part of your mind that loves drama and discord. It loves to stir up emotions and cause inner and external conflicts. Ego has a strong desire to always be right, even at the sake of your well-being! It loves to stay small and in a tiny protected comfort zone. Even if it is dangerous, familiarity is the greatest comfort to Ego. Ego is an imposter that tries to look and sound like you, except its motives and desires in life are driven only by fear. Fear is what keeps Ego alive and strong. Fear is Ego's heartbeat.

On the opposite side of fear is love. Love as previously discussed, is your Spirit. Spirit is what keeps you on the path of enlightenment. Spirit is always looking for ways to stretch and grow. It is an expanding energy, which thrives on you being authentic and true to yourself. When you are honoring your Spirit, you see the best in everything. Spirit knows that things happen to you for reasons that need to be explored, it does not try to shrink and hide. Spirit chooses to shift your perspective to see, understand and learn the valuable lessons in all life events.

It is also interesting to note, that Ego and Spirit have no concept of time—they operate on a universal structure. Therefore, events that happened decades ago have the same physiological and biological effects over your body as though it just happened. Through your memories, you relive every moment over and over again no matter how accurately or vividly your memories are. Regardless, the emotions attached to those events have the volume turned up to the max at all times when you tap into them. The good memories release hormones in your body that nourish you. Unpleasant and painful memories, release hormones that rip through your body, creating a war zone of destruction. These hormones are stress hormones, that while providing you with a surge of energy to deal with a life or death crisis, they also deplete your immune system, impair your digestive system and other organ functioning, and cause massive health and mental health issues if prolonged.

Even reading this chapter caused you to have a flood of various hormones race through you. Right from the party invitation, getting ready, anticipating who was going to be there, what you were going to say, and how you were going to act, all created emotions. Seeing the people, music, magazines, TV shows, movies, and life events that helped shape and mold you into the person you are today, caused you either happiness or sorrow. Reliving your movie reels stirred up palpable feelings you thought were long gone.

Yet, the power of being consciously aware and living through the eyes of love can help change your energy and dissolve negative thoughts no matter what you're experiencing. For example, when you chose to see your movie reel from a bird's-eye-view and took the time to understand and learn the lesson in those life events, things changed. Your thoughts started to come from a place of compassion and you immediately felt the pain and angst you were holding- begin to disappear.

Here you are, in a room with all of your images of sad moments reflecting back at you. Like the movie reel room, you have the choice to change your perspective of the event that caused you such pain. Real or imagined, internal or external, past or present, the memories you carry and the thoughts you have, create the world you choose to currently live in. You can now see that there are two sides to every event, and there is always a lesson. Choosing a different perspective will also help you shut down the flow of those destructive hormones by neutralizing that event.

Part 2: Visualization Activity

—Bird's-Eye-View

Take a bird's-eye-view to look straight down at yourself in the mirror room. You notice that you just see you. You can't see any reflections, it's you and only you. This is a good thing, because moving forward the only image that matters is the one you create in this, right here, right now, moment. In this moment, you are the one who can decide whether a happy or sad image reflects back at you.

Ego and Spirit are in a constant battle to stay in control, and because you are who they live in, you are the one who plays out their desires. One wants nothing but love and growth, the other enjoys fear and staying small. You can tell by the results that you are getting in your life as to who is winning that battle.

If you want to see a little less Ego and a lot more Spirit, keep reading. You will be introduced to concepts that will help you see how your old movie reels and mirror room images came to be, and how they are holding you back.

Part 3: Visualization Activity—Book of Life

Every now and then when you start something new in your life, you decide that you want to keep a record of the event. Think back to a time when this happened to you. Knowing that this new adventure you are about to begin is going to be epic, you decide that you want to buy a journal that will become a keepsake. You want your experience recorded in a book, with a cover that matches the feel and intensity of the journey you are about to embark on.

You head down to the bookstore filled with excitement to pick out "the" book that will forever hold the memories of this life event. You notice that there are dozens of journals to pick from. They vary in shape, size, color and weight. Even the paper inside comes in a variety of shades and textures. You had no idea that there were so many different options for a book! After touching and opening many different journals, one catches your eye. It is your favorite color and the design on the cover matches the exact energy you are feeling. As you open it up and flip the crisp, blank pages, you hear the slight crackling of the new binding. You know that binding will soften and work with you over time as you write. With a flat hand going across the page you picture your words filling the lines. As you bring the book up to your face, you inhale and take in the fresh scent of newness. You begin to get flashes of how your adventure will be played out, and you are now filled with excitement as you know this is the book that your epic journey will be recorded in. You purchase the journal and are now ready to embark on and record this exciting event.

Doesn't this adventure sound exciting and wonderful? Do you find yourself inspired to start your own journal and create a keepsake book? Do you find yourself wishing that you would have started recording events years ago? The good news is, you have!

Visualize for a moment the most beautiful book you can imagine! Picture the color of the cover and its texture. As you begin to open the book, the pages move effortlessly, as though a light breeze is blowing them. You are not sure what this magnificent book is going to be for, but you know that something this grand is clearly designed to capture something epic.

Epic indeed! This beautiful book is a detailed account of your life! You are already in the middle of a journey and have been writing and keeping track of your life events from the moment you were born! This splendid book is always with you, for it is kept in the most sacred of places. It is kept in your mind.

Picture yourself coming into this life. You are born with an open heart and mind filled with curiosity to explore and learn about this new world, and how you fit into it. You arrive without any memory or experience. To your mind, everything is new. It is blank like the pages of a new journal. For you to understand what you are learning, you need to experience it. Then, once you have that experience, you record it in the pages of your mind, or what I call your Book of Life.

The moment you started to put together your thoughts was the moment you began recording your journey and becoming the author of your life, your Book of Life. Every thought you have had, every word you have spoken and every action you have done, since coming into this world, has made it into the pages of your special and unique book.

A well written story will take you on a thrilling ride with many twists and turns. In fact, you will notice that a good author will weave together many sub stories (mini journeys) that help create the essence of the overall story. These sub stories often give you the details and clues to help understand the overall meaning to the main story. Then in the end, everything seems to come together beautifully. You are the author of your story and you create the content in your Book of Life. The difference between a best seller and your book, is that the author of the best seller is aware of what he/she is writing, which is why their book flows and makes sense. When you begin to pay attention to the events in your journey and how you are recording your experiences in the pages of your book, your life story will begin to come together, make sense and have a beautiful ending.

Let's flip back to the beginning of your book to see how your journey started, how the events in your life have been recorded, who influenced you and how the many sub stories are currently shaping your life. Remember, you are the author of your story. Once you recognize this, you can consciously edit and delete any content, in any chapter, that you no longer feel is of benefit to your overall story. Then moving forward, you can consciously choose how you want the story of your life played out.

Part 4: Visualization Activity

—Family Groove and Filters

Now, it wasn't a coincidence that the first people who you saw at the party were your parents, after all, they also had the greatest influence on creating the viewpoints you have and the behavior patterns that you carry around today.

Let's explore the complexities of your belief system by flipping back to the beginning of your Book of Life, take a stroll down memory lane and see how it all began for you.

Coming into this world, you are curious to learn who you are in relation to it. To do that, you explore your environment and start to make mental notes, which you begin to capture in your Book of Life. As you develop and notice the exciting life around you, you naturally want to expand and learn even more. You also notice that you are consistently being watched by the same people. Over time, you realize that these people are your guides. So far they have kept you safe, fed and warm. They seem like decent people, so you begin to trust them and accept them as your fearless leaders. At this point you are adjusting to life on Earth and what you are recording in your book is your experiences and observations.

Over time, you have become more aware of your environment and through experience (sometimes painful), you have learned and made note of some basic, but important, natural laws such as:

- Hot/Cold

- Up/Down

- Soft/Hard

- Light/Dark

- Tickle/Pain

- Happy/ Sad

- Sickness/Health

You are also starting to understand that the sounds coming out of your fearless leaders is actually an important language, that often matches the energy coming off of them. You realize that everything you say and do causes them to have an energetic reaction.

Sometimes, their reaction to what you do gives you warm feelings, which you learn and interpret as love. Other times, what you do, upsets and angers them, which you interpret as fear. Then, you get really confused when they aren't consistent with their reactions. One time you can do something and their reaction leaves you overflowing with love and the next time you can do the same thing, and their reaction leaves you feeling empty and cold.

You learn to adapt to all of this confusing data by a special lens that takes in your view of life. This lens, which you are born with, is unique to you. It begins as a clear, unblemished set of binoculars that allow you to examine everything, equally, in great detail, with wide-eyed wonder. But, over time, the lens becomes altered as you start adding filters. For example, you were given a filter by your parents when you were just a few pages into your journey, to help you sort all of the complex instructions coming at you. Your lens is powerful and intelligent, and with that fancy filter, it can save you time and effort and will get you where you want to go faster than if you had to process the information over each time you experienced it. Instead of having to examine and think about every emotion you experience, you can now look at it, recognize that it's already in your Book of Life, quickly tune it out, mindlessly drop it into its section and react how you "normally would."

As time marches on, you are filling up your book with all sorts of data that you accumulate through experience and instructions, and being a quick learner, you begin to see patterns such as, if I say or do this, I get a certain response. If I say or do that, I get a certain response. If I taste or touch this, I get a certain response. All of these lessons formulate into patterns that begin to shape your perception of how to get what you need and want. As you repeat these patterns, you are developing a learned behavior. Eventually, through repetition, this behavior becomes an automatic response that you don't even think about or consciously activate. Your fearless leaders did a great job of helping you make entries into your book. A couple of years in, and you have key information that guides you as you navigate your world.

Aside from your fearless leaders, whom you have learned to call parents, you have also met other interesting people who are consistently around you. You have learned to call these people grandma, grandpa, brother and sister, auntie, uncle and cousins. When you talk about them, they are called family. Some of the family you see often, others only a few times a year at events called holidays, and some, you never see at all, because they just don't fit in. All of these family members have also taught you things that you have recorded in your book. A lot of these things are very similar to what you've already learned through your parents, so you assume the information in those chapters is clearly how life must be.

The family members that are closer to your age are more fun than the older ones. You explore your environment together, and if they behave in any way different than you, you get to see what happens to them first. Sometimes, you end up laughing, sometimes crying. You can usually tell if you have been good or bad from the reaction of all the older members of your family. Being around family, especially at holidays, gives you rich material to pad your book with!

Over the years of studying and scribing the details of your family life, you begin to see predictable patterns with all of these people. You have been around and seen the same things over and over again so many times that you now just "fall into a groove". The hard work of building the groove is done, and now all you have to do is slide down the middle with ease. It took a lot of time and effort to observe, imitate, learn and become an acceptable member of the family. Everyone has their place, and everyone has learned how to exist together in what is now called: the Family Groove. As far as the family is concerned, as long as you stay inside of this groove and not try to change it, you are a good person. Wanting to be a good person, you decide you will do your best to stay inside the groove. Thankfully, you have taken in, like a wet sponge, all the data and information to keep you on track!

Remember, the Family Groove has been carved out over many generations and came to be to help protect and prepare you for surviving in the world. Like training a wild animal to exist with humans, you also have been trained and domesticated to live in the society with other humans. This training has been handed down over the generations. Your parents learned and did the best they could, based on their training from their parents, (your grandparents) as they did from their parents, and so on and so on. Everyone learns from trial and error, and over time, rules change, and everyone had to adjust their learning and training as they go.

Every human being has their own Book of Life that they have been writing since they came into existence. The early chapters in everyone's book were formed the same way yours was, which was taking in information while trying to figure out the Family Groove. You have grown to the point, where you can now step outside of the family home and begin a formal education in schools and beyond, with a "groovy" foundation to help you continue navigating this world.

Your actual view of the Family Groove is unique to you and only you can see it and understand it, as is the writing in your book. Sure, your family can relate to you, as they were the ones that inspired the first few chapters of your book and helped shape and create a Family Groove to help you interpret the world. Still, only you can truly see things as you do through your unique lens.

That special "family" filter that helped you see and sort your Family Groove is just one of the many filters from which you see the world. As you venture outside of your home, you will begin adding more filters to your lens, in hopes to keep up and make sense of this world. Every filter you add changes the view from your original unaltered lens that you entered the world with.

Part 5: Visualization Activity

—Your Comfort Zone

Human beings are designed to learn, grow and create. Like everything in nature, there is a purpose to this divine sequence. This pattern of personal evolution starts at the moment of conception and gets repeated throughout your entire lifetime, through the learning opportunities your time/space events create! As you consciously choose to step outside your comfort zone and apply the lessons from those events, you are setting off an energetic response, creating a ripple effect that impacts the world.

You spent the first nine months of your life developing in one of the most heavenly places on earth. As wonderful and as soothing as your mother's womb was, you eventually outgrew it. If you stayed longer than those nine months, you would have risked danger to you and your generous host. If you chose to stop growing too early in that gestation, you would have been at risk of dying a premature death. However, biology is genius, and you innately knew that for you to continue to learn, grow and create, you needed to break through that cozy, protective wall, at the right time in your evolution, to see what was next on your ever-evolving journey.

Sure, you felt cold and shocked at the experience of your first few moments in the world outside your nine-month miracle home, but you immediately and naturally began to adapt. You breathed in oxygen, took in nutrition and experienced life very differently, adapting, growing, and changing rapidly! Again, if you chose not to adapt, you would have died.

As graphic and harsh as that may sound, it is a natural law. This natural law is always and forever at work. If you don't adapt to life physically, emotionally and spiritually, your Life Force will shut down on different levels, leaving you at risk of death.

Let's explore your current comfort zone. Your comfort zone, like a mother's womb, keeps you safe and warm while you gather the necessary tools and information to take you on the next step of your journey. Also like a mother's womb, if you stay too long in your comfort zone, or don't adapt to your new surroundings, you will put yourself or others at a risk.

Having an understanding of your comfort zone, and becoming consciously aware of how it shows up in your life, is essential to keep you balanced and moving forward.

Let's look at how your comfort zone was formed and how it is showing up in your life. Before you can step outside of your safety circle, you need to first be aware that you are even standing in a circle.

Your parents wanted to keep you physically and emotionally safe while they taught you basic skills to navigate life. To do that, they less than consciously drew an imaginary circle around you that they felt was a safety zone. They could hear and see everything you did in that zone, and they knew that they could keep you guarded.

You, as a human, naturally wanted to explore your environment, and if you crawled outside the safety of that imaginary circle, you would be pulled back physically and emotionally. Sometimes you even got scolded or received a smack on the bottom for your adventurous ways. If you even thought about slipping past that line you knew there would be consequences for your actions and you often retreated on your own accord. Over time, you learned to stay in that imaginary safety circle and it became your home base.

As you ventured outside the safety of your home, you unconsciously brought that imaginary circle with you and you eventually became not only physically attached, but also emotionally attached to it. Whenever someone or something that seemed "scary" came too close, you turtled back into the safety of that circle.

While this tactic kept you safe as a child, it also unconsciously built you a comfort zone that has been preventing you from stepping out into the unknown and continuing the divine pattern of your personal evolution. You have, on occasion, stepped out of it when you were feeling confident. But ultimately you have been staying snug in your comfort zone with anything that challenges you emotionally, mentally, physically or spiritually.

Take a moment and think, how, when you were in your mother's womb, you naturally took the next step to grow and evolve. It's time you consciously take that natural step again.

Part 6: Visualization Activity
—Putting It All Together

You have a clear picture of how your Belief System came to be (Book of Life, Family Groove and Comfort Zone), now let's see how it grows.

You have gained many new influences and new filters outside of the family home, and from the age of five to about eighteen, they help you fill up your Book of Life pages at such a rapid rate, you can barely keep up! From sports teams, activity groups, and friends, to your religious teachings, social media, music, celebrities and school, they all form your circle of influence and have a huge impact on you and how you see the world. Meanwhile, your Family Groove is able to keep you on track and keep data properly sorted, while learning to adjust to all of the new filters being added on to your family filter.

Even though you move outside the four walls of your home and take in new data, you still mostly accept information that fits into the chapters that you already have knowledge about. Over time, these chapters grow, and the information becomes a part of you, making the domestication process complete. Everything you have recorded in your Book of Life has become your truth, not necessarily the truth of what actually is.

This is not saying what you already know is wrong. What it is saying is that unless you can look at a situation from a neutral perspective, you may be living your life based on outdated information that no longer serves and supports you. Becoming consciously aware of your experiences may give you a fresh perspective that will enhance your life. It will give you new material, outside of your Family Groove with which you can start writing new chapters.

Why is this an important skill to have? Why do you need to be able to see things differently and step outside of your Family Groove? Because, just like in the movie reel room and the room of mirrors, when you are willing to take a step back, you are able to see life from a fresh perspective. This bird's-eye-view opens up the opportunity for you to learn something new, which in return helps you stretch and grow.

Picture yourself being dropped down in the middle of Disneyland. You have a two-foot circle around you. As you slowly turn left and move your feet inch by inch, you can see so much going on around you. There are thrilling rides, fun Disney characters, wonderful looking candy shops and people having fun and laughing. As you finish your 360-degree turn, you find yourself wanting to get out to see and explore more. Just as you go to step outside of your circle, the pages of your Book of Life suddenly flip back to an earlier chapter.

You suddenly hear your mom's voice telling you that big places like this can be dangerous. You hear your dad's voice telling you the rides aren't safe. You hear your grandma's voice talking about how expensive it is, you don't have money to waste and you should 'save for a rainy day.' You stop dead in your tracks and stay standing in your little circle. After a few minutes, what looked exciting, suddenly looks scary and you no longer want to be a part of it. Staying inside of this two-foot circle is now safe and comfortable and you decide to stay put.

What happened? Why did you choose to stay in the small confined space? Unconsciously, your filter took the situation and sorted the data into experiences recorded in your past chapters. In a blink of an eye, a decision about 'now' was made based on past information.

Your filter doesn't know the reasons why you were taught things. It just knows how to sort and place the incoming data and where to pull existing data from, to help you interpret every moment of every day. You are making decisions now, as an adult, based on information you learned in your first decade of life. Remember, when you first came into this world, your parents gave you a filter so you could be safe as you began navigating the world. They did the best they could with what they knew. As did everyone who was a part of your circle of influence. You will continue to sort the information of new experiences like this until you change filters. Again, there is no right or wrong, it's just data that you have seen and filtered throughout your life. It may have served you well then, but as you have matured you are starting to get restless with some areas of your life and are perhaps wanting different results.

This truth, as you know it, can be a double-edged sword. It can either build you up and propel you forward, giving you the momentum to create an exhilarating life. Or like a machete, it can cut you down, limiting you from growing and achieving your true potential. The groove that you have built to support and protect you, can keep you on track as you navigate life or it can be the wall that is keeping you from expanding your wings.

As you grow and mature, you know the areas of your life that appear stuck, are the areas that are calling for you to view them differently. When you look at those areas from a bird's-eye-view, what you are saying is, "I'm willing to see things differently. I am wanting to expand my Book of Life and create new chapters of experience. I understand that the filter my parents gave me was to serve and protect me, but it is only one way to see things. Taking a neutral perspective is giving me the opportunity to change my filter, see events differently, learn something new and begin creating new chapters!" You have the power to write new chapters that serve and support you on your life journey.

Going back to your two-foot circle in Disneyland, see how your experience can change when you take a shifted perspective. As you slowly turn left and move your feet inch by inch, you can see so much going on around you. There are thrilling rides, fun Disney characters, wonderful looking candy shops and people having fun and laughing. As you finish your 360-degree turn, you find yourself wanting to get out to see and explore more. Just as you go to step outside of your circle, the pages of your Book of Life suddenly flip back to an earlier chapter. As you begin to hear the voices of your family chime in, you take a deep breath and choose to take a bird's-eye-view.

Like in the movie reel room, you can see everyone's perspective. You now realize that when your mom first told you that big places can be dangerous, she told you that when you were three years old at the mall, and wanted to keep you from wandering off. When you were seven years old, there was an incident at the town fair when one of the rides wasn't put together properly, causing a fatal disaster. Your dad reading this in the local paper was concerned for you, and his way to keep you safe, was warning you of the possible dangers of fair rides. Your grandma had lived through the depression and had many decades of money worries. She knew that money can fluctuate and wanted to make sure you didn't spend frivolously now, so you could experience financial security in the future.

After seeing the events from this perspective, you can see that your family was looking after you in that moment, in the best way they knew how. You can also see that not all big places are dangerous; not all rides will end in disaster; and, you won't necessarily fall into poverty by spending money. In that bird's-eye moment, you have shifted your perspective. You now understand both sides of the story, and you get to choose what information gets placed in your Book of Life. In this moment, you choose to step outside of the two-foot circle, expand your life, and enjoy all of the wonderful offerings in your "Disneyland"!

Journal Entry: Feel the Fear
and Do It Anyway
March 2011

Staying in our comfort zone is, well, comfortable. We, as humans, have developed a comfort zone for the "different areas" of our lives. For example, a person can be a daredevil in one area of their life. To them jumping out of a plane and sitting in a pit of snakes is no problem. Yet in another area of their life, telling another human being that they love them, is the most terrifying act ever. Or, how about a doctor, -who can work around blood, death, and gore but can't imagine doing something like holding a big, hairy spider.

Our comfort zone is made up of activities that we have become familiar with, and it therefore, feels comfortable. Having a comfort zone is great, but to keep growing, we need to keep expanding it. We as humans naturally expand our comfort zone in the areas of our lives where we feel confident. We also stay in a protective bubble with the areas of our lives that we are not so confident with.

We have learned to place a protective barrier around ourselves so that we don't get hurt. Think about it. If we don't step out, we won't get hurt. It just makes perfect sense! Or does it?

When we stay uncomfortably comfortable in our little bubble, we are robbing ourselves of greatness. Instead of playing the game of life to win, we are playing not to lose. We are living small and-we think we are OK with it!

Why do we do this? False Experiences Appearing Real. In other words, **FEAR.**

Our belief system is made up of a complex network of beliefs that support us, and beliefs that limit us. The beliefs that limit us from getting the positive results that we want in life are the ones that we created out of FEAR.

Somewhere along our journey we have been conditioned consciously, or less than consciously, to believe certain stories that we hear, as well as the ones we tell ourselves. Now, on the surface, these stories sound really good, and are quite believable, for both the storyteller and the one listening. However, upon closer inspection, these stories are just an excuse. An excuse to stay in our comfort zone. An excuse to not face our fears.

When it comes to taking a risk and expanding your comfort zone, does any of this self-talk ring true for you? They might not like it.

I'm not strong enough. I'll be made fun of.

I'm not good enough. Why would I do that? What if I fail?

There is no way I could do that.

I am actually OK with where I am.

This is the story that YOU tell yourself about that risk. That story is keeping you stuck in a tiny zone and keeping you from living your life fully.

So how do you know if your comfort zone is keeping you small? Well, only you know the answer. You must look at the results you are getting in your life.

For example, if you have a successful career and have no problem trying new activities but have problems with meeting a love interest, then you need to check in to the excuses that you are giving about that particular area. Ask yourself, "Am I really putting myself out there, or am I staying in my comfort zone and believing the story (FEAR) that I am telling myself."

Here is one of my FEAR stories.

I was thirty years old, had a fantastic sales job, was fit, active and had a great group of friends. However, I never had success in my love life. I dated but never really felt an emotional or spiritual connection. Then, one day I met someone. The chemistry was electric.

Everything about this person screamed, "This is the one." Yet at the same time, FEAR ripped through every fiber of my body. I wanted to retreat, run, and ignore the intense feelings I was having. I couldn't. My heart said, "This is it. Take a chance on YOU."

I listened to my heart. I stepped out and expanded my comfort zone. I was absolutely terrified. "I felt the fear and did it anyway." The fear that was racing through me, was coming to the realization that I was gay. How was I ever going to fit in to society being a lesbian? (I had some huge limiting beliefs around what being gay meant.)

I could have ignored everything that I was feeling. I could have kept telling myself lies. I could have pretended to keep being someone I wasn't. I could have lived a life void of an emotional and spiritual connection with someone. I could have stayed in a small, bubble wrapped ball. I could have let my FEAR of what society thought paralyze me from being ME. Instead, I decided to take a risk and live my life to its potential.

I am so grateful that I took that risk. Expanding my comfort zone in one area paid off in other areas! I fell in love with a woman with whom I am connected in so many ways, on so many levels. I am truly blessed to have found "the one." The other amazing thing that happened, was that by following my heart, and taking a chance, I subconsciously sent myself a message that said, "I TRUST and BELIEVE in YOU". The energy from that message flows into every other area of my life.

Now, does this mean I am done expanding my comfort zone around my sexuality? NO. I am taking another big risk and stretch right now by posting this article and announcing across the internet world that I am gay. Do I have some FEAR around it? YES, but I am feeling the fear and doing it anyway!

Remember, life is about experiencing yourself. It means that you need to continually stretch and expand your comfort zones. You will never know what greatness you have in you-until you try. When you are sitting on the "fence" of your comfort zone, seize the opportunity to grow. "Feel the fear and do it anyway." YOU are worth it.

CHAPTER 6:

Shifting Your Perspective

The moment you catch yourself thinking negative thoughts, speaking angry words, or acting in ways that are not the best version of the most brilliant vision you have of yourself, is your cue to stop and shift your perspective. Your willingness to shift your perspective is a beacon to your belief system, signifying that you are ready to learn, grow and create beyond your Ego's impulses.

There are two elements of shifting your perspective that work hand-in-hand. The first is accepting that the event is indeed neutral, and the second, is taking a bird's-eye-view. These two elements work harmoniously and at the speed of light. With practice, this life changing awareness and strategy will help create positive results in your life. That is because you are literally reprogramming your belief system! To reprogram your belief system is a willingness to look at life differently, step out of your comfort zone and expand your context of life. When you see and understand the whole picture, through your own lens, without any filters that limit you (family filter or otherwise), you can then make decisions that support you. Let's look at these in detail.

Neutral Event

As we explored in Chapter 4, as well as in my short story, a neutral event is a time/space occurrence that is specific to you and your journey through life, so you can experientially learn who you are. Your Belief System brings the positive or negative energy to the event based on previous experience.

For example, picture yourself walking down the street and a woman approaches you with her small lap dog beside her on a leash. Right now, while reading this and picturing the dog, you will have had one of the two reactions. You either caught yourself smiling at the idea of meeting the cute little dog or you were thinking who cares about the dog. Either way the **neutral event,** being the small lap dog, caused you to have either a positive or a negative reaction. This reaction is based on your previous experience with dogs or perhaps just this breed of dogs.

Every moment of everyday you are experiencing neutral events. You don't think they are neutral because you have built up super-neural highways in your brain that process and sort the data quickly and efficiently into your Book of Life at a less than conscious level. The event occurs and you react so fast that you carry on your life from a limiting perspective and you aren't even aware you are. If you catch yourself feeling fearful, angry or hateful, that is your cue to pay attention and Shift Your Perspective (SYP).

Now that you have slowed your thinking process down enough to recognize that you are indeed experiencing a neutral event, you can now flow into the second element which is taking a "bird's-eye-view".

Bird's-Eye-View

The bird's-eye-view occurs when you cross over into the Soul Games and begin to see that there are two sides to the coin. Like in my short story, you can now visualize and understand that there is more to the event than just your viewpoint. This is a place of personal power. When you take this viewpoint, you are willing to see the whole picture and challenge your existing belief system. Doing this, will give you the choice to respond to the situation instead of just reacting.

Imagine yourself walking down the block in your neighborhood and seeing a big number 6 painted on the sidewalk. As you are pondering the significance of this number, your neighbor approaches from the opposite way and stops and looks down at what you're staring at. After a few seconds he looks up and asks, "What do you suppose is the significance of this number 9?"

Looking stunned at your neighbor, because clearly the number is a 6, you decide before you ask what planet is he on, you pause and take a bird's-eye-view of the situation. In your mind's eye, you are like an eagle flying overhead looking down and now you can see the entire picture, not just your viewpoint. You realize that from where he is standing, he does indeed see a 9! You are both correct! Instead of having an I'm right and you are wrong conversation, you both put your heads together to see what the significance of what either a 6 or a 9 is doing painted on your sidewalk.

Taking a bird's-eye-view will change how you respond to a situation. The neat part is, it doesn't have to be a "live" event you are experiencing-it can be done with a past experience as well. Going back to the small dog example, you remember when you were seven years old, running up to the dog and as you reached to pet the dog, it snapped at you. Upset and scared you ran home and from that moment on, you have been afraid of dogs. Now, taking a bird's-eye-view of that moment, see yourself as that little girl running up to the dog. What you didn't see then but you do now, is the owner, who was a frail senior citizen, couldn't stop or warn you in time, to not pet her dog on top of the head. You took off too fast for the owner to catch you and let you know that the dog is really friendly. But, with the dog being blind, you need to let him sniff you first.

Now that you see the whole picture, you can begin asking yourself questions that get you seeing the situation from both sides of the coin. Such as, do I still actually feel this way, or is it energy from when I was seven years old? How is being afraid of dogs supporting me? How is it limiting me? How can I respond differently, now that I realize that not all dogs are mean or vicious, that they will sometimes nip at people when they are scared or hurt? This one fundamental shift in your awareness now opens up the opportunity for you to begin having a relationship with dogs instead of living in fear of them.

In summary, Shifting Your Perspective (SYP) is a two part awareness strategy that puts you in the driver's seat of the choices you choose to make. When you begin looking at past events in your life and current events from this perspective, you open up your context and challenge your belief system. You are truly operating from a place of personal power!

Workplace Example

I worked as a sales rep for a convenience and packaged goods company and sold products and displays into grocery stores. A large part of my job was to sell in bookings, where stores got a price break to help plan for upcoming flyer features. For the most part, my customers were open and willing to listen to me and participate in these sales opportunities. However, I did have one account that was impossible to deal with. I could not get them to engage in anything I presented. They would literally throw the product booking forms onto the floor without even looking at them! I would feel myself getting angry for being treated so poorly and I would leave the store frustrated, and that energy often carried over into the rest of my day. Being that I was an employee, I couldn't just skip this account, it was my job to make it work. Based on the results I was getting, clearly, I was missing the mark with this account.

I was meditating on my dynamics with that store and its management one morning and had a thought. Perhaps they aren't engaging with me because I am not presenting in a way that speaks to them. I knew I had to shift my perspective. The store manager's reaction to my bookings was just a neutral event. I was bringing the energy to my frustrations based on what I believed was an acceptable response, which would be for the store manager to take a moment and look at the booking. I did a bird's-eye-view, looked at the big picture and spent time trying to understand the event from his perspective, the other side of the coin.

This is what I was able to see and understand:

- They are a decades old, family run, small-town store.

- They made their best profits when they could negotiate with the sales reps.

- Product used to be delivered straight from the vendor to the store. Now it goes through the banner warehouse and savings don't necessarily get passed down to the stores.

- They believe that they can still negotiate a deal with the reps.

- Reps that don't play ball with them, clearly aren't worth supporting.

- They are frustrated because they can't keep up and take losses like the bigger box store can.

SYP helped me see the bigger picture. On my next sales trip into the store, I asked questions and talked to them about the "good old days", and asked them how the "new" direction that their head office was using to deal with vendors was affecting their business. Ten minutes later, I was still listening to the store manager recall how amazing business was five years earlier and, how now, they can't make a profit anymore. The understanding I gained from a fresh perspective helped me speak to the store manager in a language he could understand. Our relationship changed after that. Even though he still didn't do bookings with me, as I had no control over pricing, we did develop an amicable relationship. He no longer threw my bookings on the floor, and I never left his store angry or frustrated.

The beauty of shifting your perspective is that you begin to consciously build up knowledge that you can apply to other situations you face in life. You are creating new material, based on your conscious experience to go into your Book of Life. Our hardest times will often lead us to our greatest growth. I became a better sales rep because of that customer. By shifting my perspective, seeing the big picture, and not taking his response personally, I was able to engage that store manager. After that, whenever I met with my small town stores, I came from that shifted perspective and my relationships flourished. I took what I perceived to be a crappy situation and consciously responded with a Warrior Mindset and it made a fundamental difference in that area of my life.

As an additional bonus, when you shift your perspective on a past event, where you don't have all of the facts, such as the experience of facing the small dog as a seven-year-old, what you are actually getting to do is make up a possible story that demonstrates the other side of the coin. Even though what you make up is not necessarily accurate, taking time to ponder the event and imagining that the dog was scared and blind, has now given you a new perspective that has now lessened your fear of dogs. You are starting to consciously change old material in your Book of Life that is no longer serving you and replace it with information that is more relevant to where you are now in life.

Journal Entry: Rose Colored Glasses
January 2011

The first time I heard the expression "take off your rose-colored glasses" I was probably 15. I was perplexed because I clearly didn't have any glasses on. So, when I got home, I immediately asked my mom what the heck that meant. "Well," she said, "It means the person is seeing things from the sunny side. Even in the middle of a crisis, they don't see the problem."

That sounded pretty good to me. Why would someone want me to take those off? Then my mom finished her sentence. "To the point that they annoy the other person. Their head is so far in the clouds that they don't see reality." Hmmm.

As I have grown with and studied personal development, I have learned that chastising people for their "rose-colored" glasses is a HUGE mistake, and here is why.

I have a thing for sunglasses with a polarized lens. The world appears to look even better with them on. I have several pairs because each has a unique lens that filters differently, depending on the light conditions. For example, I have a pair with an orange lens that works best on overcast days with flat light. Somehow, the world seems brighter and things just "pop" out with them on. If people ask me about them, I always give them an enthusiastic spiel about how much better the world looks. And I excitedly offer them the opportunity to try them on, which they eagerly do. Quite often, I will try theirs on as well to compare the differences.

When people enjoy their sunglasses, they often will encourage other people to try them on. "You should see how awesome things look with these," they say. Without hesitation we often try them on. Sometimes, the world does look better through them. Sometimes, it looks the same or not as good as it did with our glasses. (This makes us excited because it confirms that we do indeed have a great pair of sunglasses.) When people are into it, they have their glasses in one hand and yours in the other, and they switch back and forth to "really" see the differences.

We, as humans literally look at everything we see in life through the filter of OUR belief system. If other people's "filters" aren't the same as ours, then they must be wrong. We never really step into the other person's shoes and give their point of view a chance.

We are so willing to look at the world through another person's sunglasses and acknowledge that their lens may be different and possibly even a little better than our sunglass lens. Yet we have trouble seeing life through their eyes and accepting that they may see things a little different from us.

Being able to put your beliefs aside to "see and understand" another's point of view, is giving yourself the opportunity to see the world through a different filter. (What a gift!) You never know, that filter may help you see things from a whole new perspective. Seeing things in a different light may then help you discover solutions instead of problems. Remember, you don't know the quality of your lens, until you can compare it to someone else's lens.

The next time you find yourself questioning someone's point of view, take a moment to "really see" where they are coming from. Depending on the light, "rose-colored glasses" may be a good lens for you to try on.

CHAPTER 7:

Rise Up

I introduced you to the Soul Games and Belief System Cycle in Chapters 2 and 4. Now, you are going to learn how these two systems come together with a process I created and call "Rise Up."

Rise Up is an awareness strategy that bridges your current belief system to the source that is creating it. This awareness opens up the opportunity for you to see the bigger picture, which gives you the space to examine the data in your Book of Life, and then make new and empowering decisions, based on updated information that serves and supports you.

I have been asked time and again, how is it that I have such a calm, positive attitude around death and dying such as my diving experience in Cozumel. Why was I able to get through breast cancer without having complete melt downs? The answer is simple. I was instinctively doing the process that I now call Rise Up.

It starts at what I call the "Critical Junction". The Critical Junction is "the" moment when you pay attention to your thoughts and feelings and immediately pause your Belief System Cycle, shift your perspective and cross over into the Soul Games. Once crossed over into the Soul Games, from your bird's-eye-view, you can look down and determine your mindset, based on your current thoughts and feelings. Are you coming from a state of empowerment (love) or from a state of suffering (fear)? Are you being driven by Spirit or Ego?

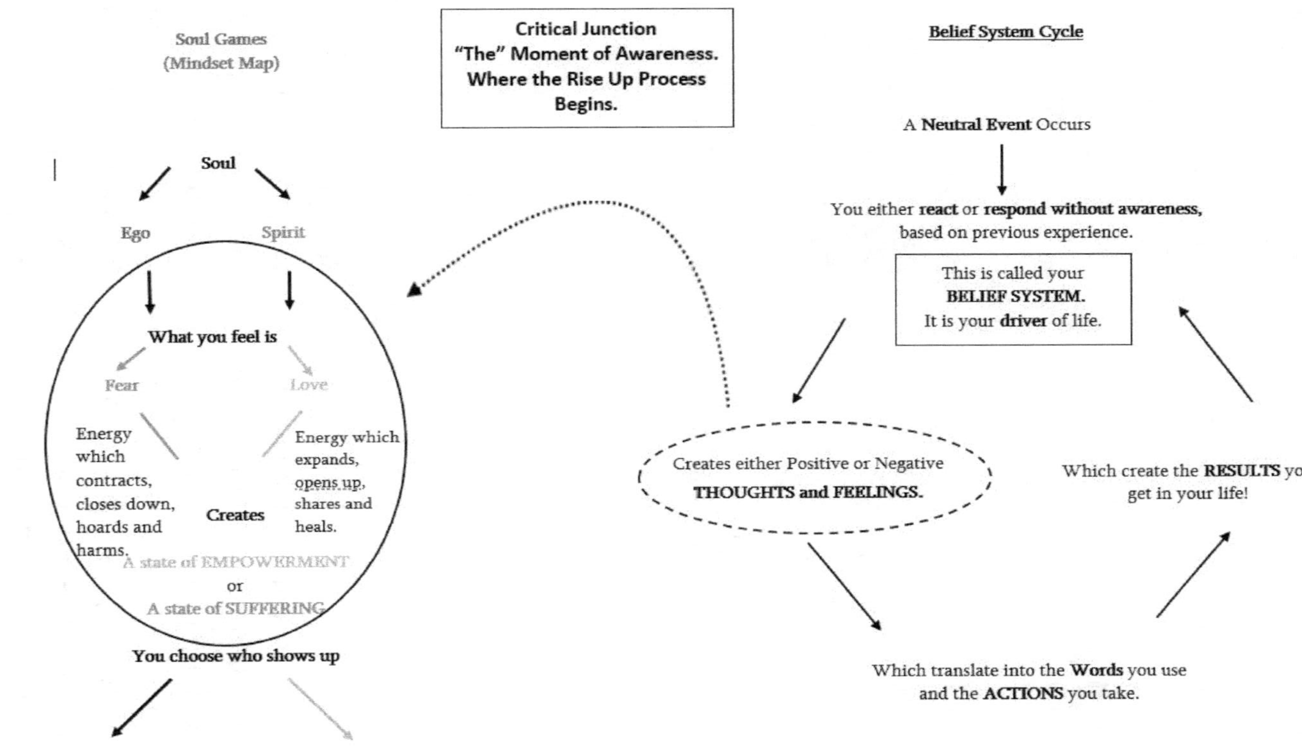
Soul Games
(Mindset Map)

Critical Junction
"The" Moment of Awareness.
Where the Rise Up Process Begins.

Belief System Cycle

A Neutral Event Occurs

Soul

Ego

Spirit

You either react or respond without awareness, based on previous experience.

What you feel is

This is called your BELIEF SYSTEM. It is your driver of life.

Fear

Love

Energy which contracts, closes down, hoards and harms.

Energy which expands, opens up, shares and heals.

Creates

Creates either Positive or Negative THOUGHTS and FEELINGS.

Which create the RESULTS you get in your life!

A state of EMPOWERMENT
or
A state of SUFFERING

You choose who shows up

Which translate into the Words you use and the ACTIONS you take.

From this eye in the sky perspective, you also get to see the event from both sides of the coin. After doing some Big Picture Processing (answering specific questions that help you visualize living your life from both sides of the coin), you get to consciously choose which side is more aligned with who you are and who you want to be in relation to the event. You are now making decisions based on beliefs created by you, in a conscious state of being.

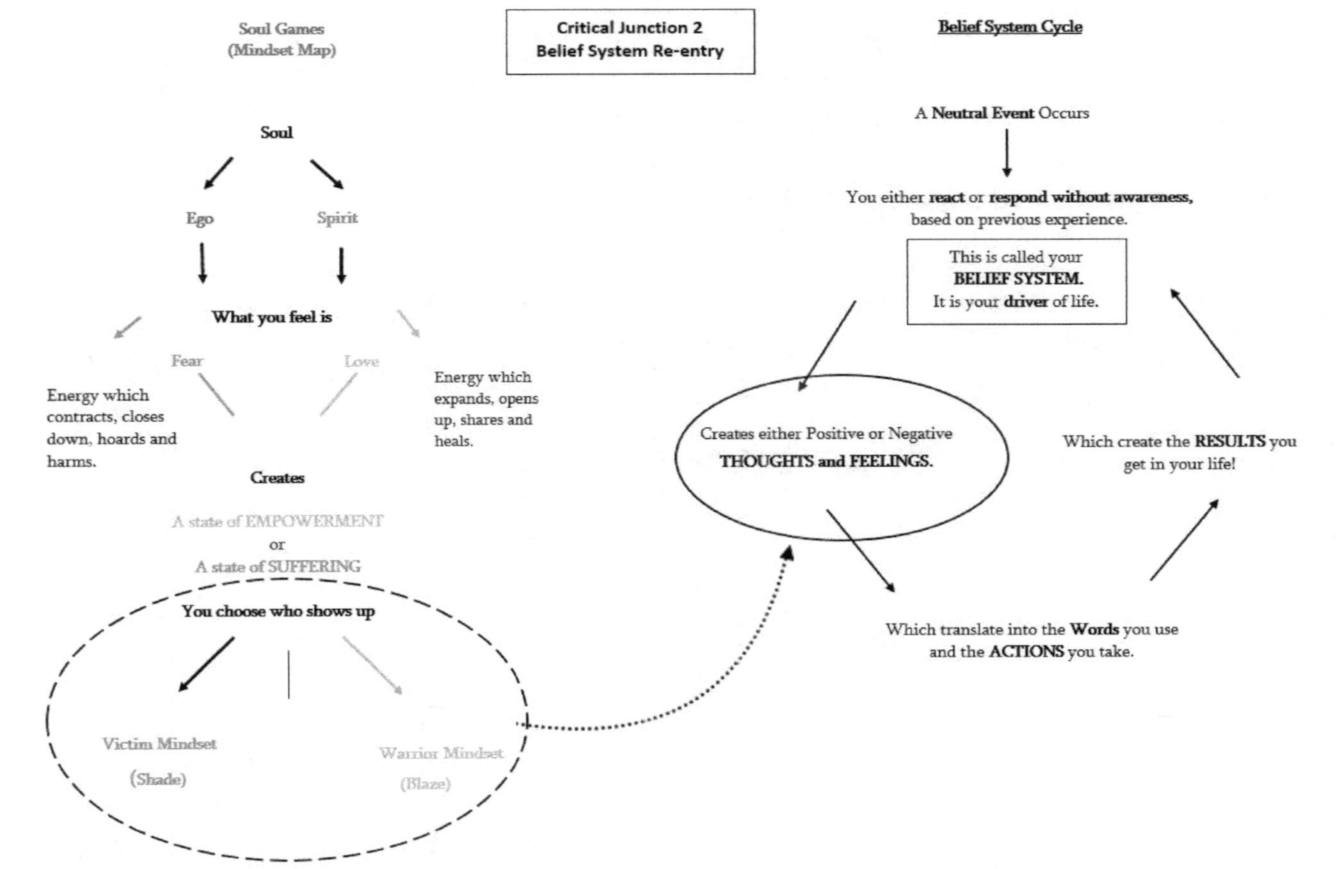
Soul Games
(Mindset Map)

Critical Junction 2
Belief System Re-entry

Belief System Cycle

Soul

Ego

Spirit

What you feel is

Fear

Love

Energy which contracts, closes down, hoards and harms.

Energy which expands, opens up, shares and heals.

Creates

A state of EMPOWERMENT
or
A state of SUFFERING

You choose who shows up

Victim Mindset
(Shade)

Warrior Mindset
(Blaze)

A Neutral Event Occurs

You either react or respond without awareness, based on previous experience.

This is called your BELIEF SYSTEM. It is your driver of life.

Creates either Positive or Negative THOUGHTS and FEELINGS.

Which translate into the Words you use and the ACTIONS you take.

Which create the RESULTS you get in your life!

Whichever mindset you choose to re-enter the Belief System Cycle with, is perfectly fine. If you decide after doing your Big Picture Processing, that sitting in a Victim Mindset with your current limiting beliefs is where you need to be, that is okay. There will come a time when staying constricted and small doesn't serve you anymore. You will, once again feel that awareness to pause your Belief System Cycle and cross over into the Soul Games, where you will once again get the opportunity to choose whichever mindset you want to show up with.

You will always and forever have the opportunity to learn, grow and create from the experiences of your events throughout your lifetime. Your life exists of time/space events just for you to experientially know who you are. You are the creator of your life and have the personal power to choose your thoughts, words and actions to each and every one of these events. Remember events are neutral, you are the one bringing the energy to it based on your belief system, which you now understand and have the power to "rise up" and change.

CHAPTER 8:

New Diagnosis Story

You now know that your cancer diagnosis was a neutral event. You brought the energy to it based on past experience. You were reacting from data filed away in your Book of Life. This data was originally someone else's opinion that became your reality, and it became a part of your belief system. Being the great author you are, you have the power to erase old, outdated information and re-write those chapters with data that is more in alignment with who you are now.

So, let's go back in time to when you were first getting your diagnosis. This time though you will focus on your reaction when the doctor informed you that you have breast cancer. The majority of women will react in shock, disbelief and even displaced anger. If you fall into this majority, that is normal. Your reaction is your cue to pause and pay attention to where in the Belief System Cycle you are and remind yourself that getting your diagnosis is just a neutral event. In that split second of awareness feel yourself rise up. You are now experiencing the **"Critical Junction."** You have become aware of your thoughts and feelings and are now crossing over into the **Soul Games with a bird's-eye-view.**

To get a clear picture of why you reacted the way you did to your diagnosis, you need to determine why your belief system is coming from fear. Take a moment and reflect back on all of your memories, visions and experiences you have had about cancer throughout your lifetime. These could come from the conversations you heard your parents having, television shows and movies. You may have been witness to someone you know who had cancer. Whatever your experience of cancer has been so far, has become the filter of how you view and understand all cancer, whether it is accurate or not.

As you begin to understand why your belief system defaulted to fear, you can consciously change your thoughts about it. You can determine if the info in your Book of Life is supporting or limiting you. When you begin questioning the motives of your Ego, you become more open to the whispers of your Spirit. This opening allows you to do Big Picture Processing (BPP) and ask deeper questions that give you an even greater understanding of the event from both sides of the coin.

These are the BPP questions I intuitively asked myself through each and every leg of my climb.

- What two words describe how I feel right now?

- What is the worst-case scenario? What will my life look like if I have to travel down this road?

- What is the best-case scenario? What will my life look like if I have to travel down this road?

- Who do I want to be in relation to what I am experiencing here and now?

- What am I grateful for?

Doing Big Picture Processing will deepen the space for you to really tune into the frequency of Spirit, listen to its wisdom and experience perspective from the other side of the coin. Instead of just being pulled around by fear, you will also be divinely guided by love. The awakening is complete! You now get to choose the mindset you want to experience this neutral, time/space event with. You decide who you want to be in relation to the event. You decide if you want to listen to Ego or to Spirit. You get to choose if you want to show up with a Victim Mindset or a Warrior Mindset.

Stop right now and journal your cancer diagnosis story again, this time from a shifted perspective. When you are done, create another list of words that describe how you feel right now. When you are done, place this list beside the other list from the first time you journaled your diagnosis story.

Here is the most brilliant part about shifting your perspective on a past event. Even though the event is long over, your mind doesn't know the difference! You can re-tell your story from a fresh perspective and your mind and body will react as though it is happening now. This gives you the personal power to reframe any negative energy you were unconsciously carrying around, into positive energy that you can consciously tap into and assist you on your life journey.

Whether your stories are real or imagined, if they happen internally (stories you tell yourself) or externally (voicing your beliefs out loud), they are just your experiences based on the information that you had at that time. Re-examining them from a shifted perspective is a spiritual and emotional "do over" for you.

CHAPTER 9:

Opposites

There is no right or wrong way to go through breast cancer. As I talked about in chapter 1, your journey is your experience, and whatever image is on the cover of your box, is your puzzle to figure out. The universe has been intelligently designed to give you dualities so you can experientially learn who you are in relationship to the world. You wouldn't know yourself as happy unless you experienced sadness. You wouldn't know yourself as healthy unless you experienced sickness. You would not understand life without death. As you journey up the Pink Mountain, you will be facing many situations that will put you in a state of suffering whether that be physical, mental, emotional or spiritual. Your Ego will be turned up high causing fear to take over your being. When you catch yourself in a state of suffering, with a Victim Mindset, enduring your darkest moments, remember, there is an opposite. There will always be an opposite. You just have to be in the game. Keep your feet moving, keep your faith and trust the intelligence of the universe. You have the power to shift your perspective, look at both sides of the coin, challenge your Ego and look for the light of Spirit. You can choose a Warrior Mindset and choose to be in a state of empowerment.

Every moment of every day, your time/space events will keep you moving back and forth between opposites, so you can experientially know who you are. Let's explore this concept using a swing analogy.

Chances are the first time you experienced a swing was at the park or in the back yard. You probably don't really remember, but the only way you could get moving was if your parents, family, friend, or relative gave you a push. Your swing took you way up high and you felt a calmness as you hit what seemed like the top of world. Then, a moment later you felt your body retreating down and backwards, then up to the complete opposite side. As you paused at the top of the backswing, you almost felt like you were going to plummet straight down into the ground. In fact, your tummy tickled with fear. After a few pushes your body started adapting to the sensations and soon you were moving mindlessly back and forth until your parents stopped pushing you.

As you grew, your parents taught you how to use the swing on your own. You would run to the swing set, hop on the seat and start pumping your legs. After a few determined pumps, you started to build momentum and the next thing you knew you were enjoying the thrilling ride that the swing gave you. Both the ups and down were fun, although admittedly, on the downswing your tummy would get nervous butterflies. They were always fluttering, almost like a warning to keep you safe. To not appear scared, you kept going and eventually, you got used to it. Even though you were getting braver riding the swing, you weren't quite as brave as the older kids who dismounted their swings midair.

After a couple of years of swing time you got stronger, and braver and you were now big enough to try your mid-air dismount. As you got your swing rocking back and forth, you decided to go for your dismount. As you let go of the chains, you plummeted face first to the ground. You were hurt and quite shaken up. Dusting yourself off, you looked around stunned, wondering where you went wrong. That's when you noticed that the kids landing their dismount were letting go on the upswing, not the downswing. You got back on the swing, but you were too scared to get your legs pumping. You were just sitting there, not moving. After a few minutes, other kids came by and commented that if you weren't going to use the swing, you should just get off of it. Feeling a little embarrassed, you decided that the swing just wasn't for you.

Walking away you turned around and took one last look at all of the other kids playing on the swings. Some were laughing, some were screaming, some were being supported by their parents, some were making it happen on their own, and others were flying through the air and landing that perfect dismount and smiling. Watching all of the fun and commotion, you decided that you didn't want to miss out. Walking away from all of the thrills the swing provides, because of one messy dismount, suddenly seemed ridiculous. Adamant that you weren't going to miss out on one more moment of ride time, you marched back to the swing, hopped up on the seat and began pumping your legs with renewed energy. In mere moments, you were swinging up high and almost touching the sky, then back down, through and up high on the scary side. You were a little nervous on the "scary" side but you hung on, took a deep breath and before you knew it, you were back down and on your way up towards the sun again.

After a few minutes of moving through the exhilarating extremes of your swing ride, you decide that it was time to try your mid-air dismount. As you started coming down from the back swing, you took a deep breath and as soon as you felt yourself hit the upswing you let go. You were literally flying through the air! You felt as free as a bird, even if it was for just a second. You saw the ground coming in fast and you softened your knees to prepare yourself for your landing. You felt one foot touch the ground and then the other and knew you nailed your dismount. You sprung up hollering in delight at what you just did. With a renewed excitement, you immediately got back up on the swing again feeling thankful that you never walked away from the failure of your first attempt.

As you move back and forth and between a Warrior and Victim Mindset, know that you will fall down, you will feel pain and you will feel fear, and that is okay. You need to experience all of the darkness so you can truly understand how glorious the opposite is. The key to successfully figuring out your soul's true passion and purpose, is to stay on the swing and learn. Learn all you can, continue to grow and create until you place your final piece of the puzzle.

Now that you have both lists of your thoughts and feelings from your diagnosis stories in front of you, place your original list on the left and your new list on the right. Imagine yourself sitting in the middle. Know that just like the swing, you will be going back and forth between the two extremes. With self-awareness, you get to determine which side you want to be on. If you need to sit in the darkness of shade that is fine, you need to experience what you need to experience. The moment you decide you don't like the feelings of that downswing, know that you have the power to shift your perspective and move to the upswing and lightness of Blaze. There is no right or wrong way to swing. Embrace the entire experience, both the butterflies of Shade and the calmness of Blaze.

CHAPTER 10: Web of Life

Spider Web

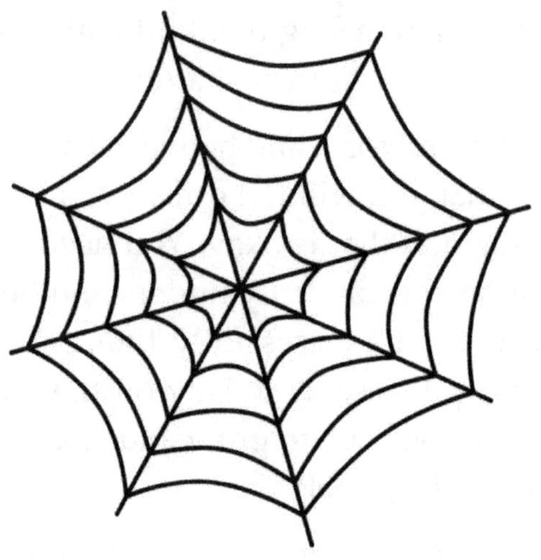

Look at this spider web with its perfect design. It has sections built in to give it proper strength and flexibility. If you notice, there are fine threads that connect each section- so that when the spider is sitting in one part of the web, she can feel what is going on in another. This helps protect her as well as signaling to her that she has food. If, for any reason a part of the web gets destroyed, whether that be from a predator, man or otherwise, the spider will immediately go out and fix the section that was affected. She knows that having even one part of her web down will have a negative impact on her life. She takes accountability for the entire web, no matter who or what has interfered or destroyed it. She doesn't lay blame and she doesn't become self-righteous, she intuitively knows that it is up to her to accept what is and fix it. She knows her existence in life depends on it. The spider, by nature, always has the mindset of a warrior. She doesn't have a belief system that has been influenced by others, nor does she have an Ego trying to run the show. She is just being a spider and acting in the laws of nature.

Picture each of your life areas being a section of the spider web. Even though you view your life areas as separate from each other, you can clearly see how intertwined they are. If one section is dysfunctional in any way, it will impact the other areas.

Spider Web and You

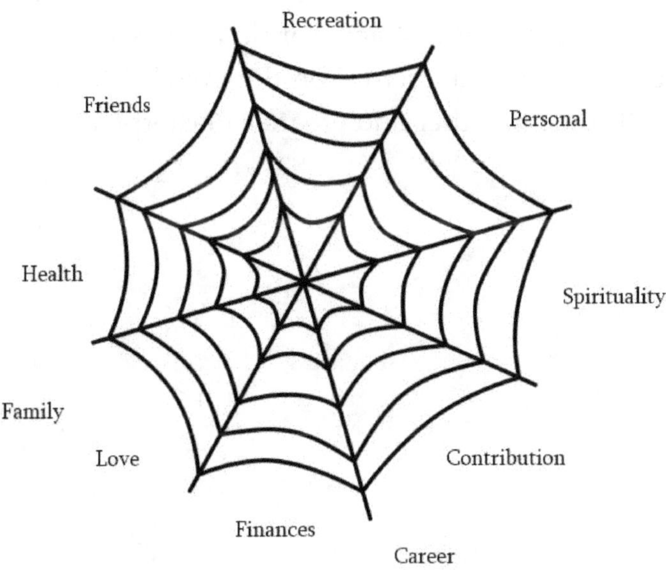

Breast cancer has come along and plunked itself down pretty hard in the health section of your web. You can clearly see how this has caused a disturbance and is impacting your entire web. You can't change that breast cancer has landed in your life, but like the spider, you can choose to respond to it in a way that allows you to be in control of the impact it has on you and the important things around you.

Take a moment and think about some of the major events you have experienced over your life. I'm sure you have had many things come crashing into your web over the years. Regardless of which life area the event began in, the energy and vibration of that event spilled across the entire web. If you were to zoom in and take a micro-view of your Web of Life, all you would see and feel is chaos. When you are caught up in the web, everything appears and feels disconnected and separate. Yet, if you were to step back and take a macro-view of the web, you would see the intelligence and the beauty of the design and having breast cancer is just another time/space event that adds to that design. Like the picture on the puzzle box, all the little pieces will come together and create a masterpiece.

Web of Life

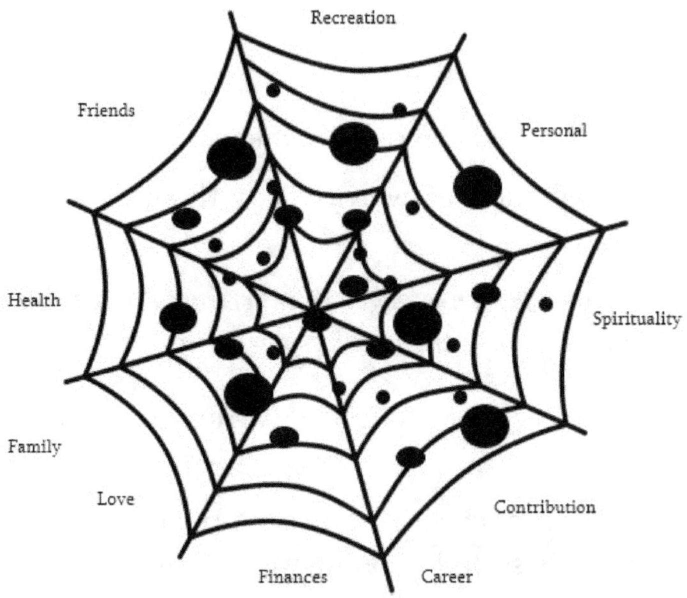

You now have the tools to help you shift your mindset, the moment you feel a disturbance in your web. Have faith that your soul knows what it is doing. Like the spider intuitively maintaining her web, regardless of the events that come into play for her, you too need to trust what is coming into play for you. You have been victimized by breast cancer, but you do not have to be a victim. Choose a warrior mindset, maintain your web and enjoy the precious time you have, however long it may be.

CHAPTER 11:

You Are a Warrior

What do you think when you hear the word warrior?

This is the definition of warrior as written in the Webster dictionary.

> ***Warrior**-a person engaged or experienced in warfare*
> ***Broadly**-a person engaged in some struggle or conflict*

While the above is true, I believe a warrior is so much more. It is…

• A woman who chooses to rise up and challenge the situation, regardless of the conditions in front of her.

• A woman who recognizes the value she has to offer the world and makes it her mission to bring it to life and make a difference in the world around her.

• A woman who knows that every challenge is not a battle to shame the loser, but a battle to personally evolve.

• A woman who knows that if she has a heartbeat, she still has purpose.

• A woman who sees the blessing in every event.

• A woman who can accept the event as is and choose how she wants to respond to it.

• A woman who chooses to empower herself and her Life Force.

• A woman who looks fear in the eye and chooses to keep her feet moving forward.

• A woman who listens to her body, her inner wisdom and chooses to honor what it needs.

• A woman who will reach out and lend a hand when needed and equally as important, will reach out and accept a hand when she needs it.

• A woman who chooses to rediscover her inner strength and chooses to Thrive the Climb!

A warrior means different things to different people. I encourage you to take a moment to add to this list or create and write down your own definition of a warrior. The biggest takeaway of this moment is for you to recognize who it is you are reading about and describing. I hope you truly feel that you are the essence in these words. The more connected you are to your inner warrior, the easier she will be to find during your hardest times.

CHAPTER 12:
Climbing Strategies

Like any climb, applying strategies from those who have gone before, can make a huge difference as you head up the mountain for the first time. These strategies will help you stay empowered throughout your journey.

Journaling

One of the most important pieces of equipment to carry with you is a journal. You will be overflowing with a lot of emotions through every step and leg of this climb, and journaling will give you an outlet. If you write and express the emotions you are feeling, negative energy will be released and positive energy will be harnessed.

Any fear-based energy you are consciously aware of, needs to be let out. You do not want that manifesting inside of you. Remember Shade loves fear and drama and will do anything to keep you small and scared. You have the personal power to release it. But, before you can release it, you need to recognize that you are holding it. You can't put something down unless you know you are holding it.

The more you write, the more you become in tune with yourself. You will start to notice where in your Belief System Cycle you sitting by the words you use to describe the events, as well as, the words you use to describe yourself. Journaling is a way to check in to see if you are being influenced by Shade or Blaze. The words you use attach meaning to your experience. Language is reflective of what you think and believe. (Belief System Cycle in chapter 4)

Remember, thoughts are the first level of creation. Words describe what you are thinking, and action is your words in motion.

For example, using healthy eating as a neutral event

A Victim Mindset would go something like this:

Thought: "Every time I try to make diet changes, I fail."

Words: "I can't stick to anything. Maybe it will be different this time, but I doubt it."

Action: Stopping at a fast food restaurant for dinner.

A Warrior Mindset would go something like this:

Thought: "When I eat well, I feel so good."

Words: "I will be successful this time because I want to be healthy."

Action: Planning meals ahead of time and having healthy food ready.

Here is a sample list of some common thoughts and words that will either deflate you or lift you up.

Negative: I can't, I wish, I have to, I had no choice, Maybe, I'll try, It's not fair

Positive: I can, I will, I know, I choose to, I enjoy, I want to

Begin to pay attention to the words you use. If you are not enjoying the destination your words are taking you to, you have the power to shift your perspective and change them.

Affirmations

As you have been learning, your belief system shapes the way you see and interpret the world. Changing your beliefs can happen in one of the two ways. One way is a dramatic, life altering event. The other way is through conscious repetition and reinforcement. I personally like the latter, as it actually helps to re-program the neural highways in your brain creating longer lasting and hopefully permanent change. However, if you are reading this book, you are also experiencing the former. Now is truly the time for you to stretch yourself, examine your beliefs and create the positive energy you want in your life.

A fantastic way to start getting into the groove of mindful writing is to create affirmations.

Why Affirmations? It is a seed of positive intention which you plant in 'here and now' that will grow (as long as it's nurtured and fed). An affirmation is a statement of assertion that something is already so. Real or imagined, as long as you repeat it, your brain will think it.

The sky is the limit when it comes to writing your affirmations. The most empowering and effective affirmations contain the 4 P's.

Personalized (They should always say "I" and your name.)
Present tense (They should say "I" and your name "am".)
Positive

Passionate (Your passion is essential yet comes from how you state the affirmation to yourself.)

Here are examples of some affirmations I created back in 2009 and still use today.

I, Cindy, am a smart, confident, powerful loving woman.

I, Cindy, have a strong, fit, healthy, vibrant body from which I positively impact the world.

I, Cindy, give and receive love openly and freely.

I, Cindy, see the beauty and gifts in the people around me.

If you have a disconnection saying your affirmation because you don't yet believe it for yourself, you can alter it by saying you are in the process of…

I, Cindy, am in the process of becoming a smart, confident, powerful loving woman.

I, Cindy, am in the process of having a strong, fit healthy, vibrant body from which I positively impact the world.

I, Cindy, am in the process of giving and receiving love openly and freely.

Habits are formed through daily practice or reinforcement, and reprogramming your brain happens the same way. Through repetition, your affirmations will begin to create new neural highways in your brain and over time you will believe what you are saying and will begin to see evidence of it coming true in your life.

Solidify the Power of Affirmations NOW

To help solidify the power of affirmations for you, I created a FREE downloadable guide and video to help you incorporate this into your daily empowerment ritual.

Get the Breast Cancer Affirmation Writing Guide here.

Create the person you want to be as you thrive through breast cancer.

https://thrivetheclimb.com/free-affirmations

Meditation

There are many different studies and written accounts on the positive effects of meditation. I, for one, am a big fan. If you have never meditated before, you might get some resistance from your monkey mind. In other words, your Ego is going to try and interrupt any attempts at you making an effort to connect with your Spirit. Heck, that little bugger likes to get in the way no matter how much experience you have sitting on the pillow. Don't feel bad about her showing up, that is her job. The more you can learn how to consciously shut Shade down, you will begin to do it on a less than conscious level as well.

For the record, you don't have to sit cross legged on a pillow to meditate. I personally sit in my lazy boy chair, as my legs and back don't like being a pretzel. The last time I was able to sit cross legged was in grade one! Bottom line, you sit however makes you comfortable. The key is to be relaxed so you can breathe and start clearing your mind.

I actually started meditating by memorizing and repeating my affirmation statements. Over time, I added more of them and eventually I created quite a routine. Two years ago, I had the opportunity to do Seduction of Spirit with Deepak Chopra. That elevated my practice to a whole other level. In the ten years that I have been meditating, I have built up a tool box of different routines that vary in length of time. This way, regardless of where I am or how much time I have, I can still take a moment to connect with my Spirit.

Exercise

If you have been active up to your point of diagnosis, I would encourage you to maintain your exercise program as much as you can. The compounding effects of cancer treatment do catch up to you, that is why it's important to listen to your body and not overdo it. The first couple of rounds of chemo, I was still able to ride the exercise bike and do strength training, albeit my intensity and duration dropped, but I still made an effort. By the fourth chemo, my energy levels changed quite a bit. Doing my exercise routine became a struggle. Instead of abandoning fitness completely, I accepted that a daily walk to the dog park was the best I could do and that is what I did. I knew that it was important to keep my body moving. Becoming sedentary would cause my body to shut right down and I didn't want that.

Now, if you were sedentary at the time of your diagnosis, I would encourage you to at least get out and walk. There have been more and more studies coming out that demonstrate the benefits of exercise for cancer patients. I was lucky and was able to participate in a Yoga class for people going through cancer, and it had a tremendous impact on my health and wellbeing. I would highly recommend talking to your doctor, or the medical professionals at your cancer centre, and see what you can do to add some movement to your day.

Books on Spirituality

(Or any kind of reading that brings you feelings of peace)

The other positive habit I set in motion 10 years ago, and still do today, is to read something positive and uplifting for a minimum of twenty minutes in the morning. I find this helps to set my tone for the day. If you combine reading with your meditation routine, you will be starting the day with an energy and clarity that will help keep Ego in line!

Reading books written by authors that you feel a connection to is like having your own personal advisor and cheerleader whenever you need it. I have some books that I have read countless times, and every time I read them, I pull out new nuggets of gold that seem to resonate with whatever my current needs are. Each time I read these books, again and again, they have a unique and positive impact on my life. So, don't dismiss a book you love just because you've read it before. If it's "calling to you", pick it up and re-visit your old friend. It might have something else to teach you or a new way to comfort you this time.

Music Therapy

This is one of my favorites! Music literally lights me up! In fact, I will share this little blog post I wrote to help inspire you to invite music into your journey:

Journal Entry: Music Motivates
(2011)

I love music. I always have, I always will. Music is a pure form of motivation. It can reach deep inside of me and wake me up on so many levels and move me physically and mentally. It inspires me to get up, move and achieve my goals. With the right beat, I can't help but get up and bust some moves. It doesn't matter where or when, if the music is playing, I will shake it. I have a fridge magnet that says, "Dance like no one is watching," and I do make that my motto. I love how free I feel when I let the music move me. We, as humans are meant to feel the energy and vibration of music. Ask yourself what music moves and inspires you to step it up and move in life.

I love connecting to a song. If I relate to the lyrics of a song, I find that I never get tired of listening to it. It is almost like the artist is singing to me with my words and feelings (somebody actually understands and gets me!). Roberta Flack brought that concept to life for us in the 70's with her song "Killing Me Softly". Although, I do have to admit, the first time I heard it, was when the Fugees covered it in the 90's.

Right now, I am listening to Melissa Etheridge. She is a true singer/songwriter. I have really connected with her new CD, Fearless Love. The lyrics in many of these songs mirror the journey that I am on right now (at least that is how I interpret them). When I first heard her lyrics, I was blown away. The beliefs and concepts that Melissa has put to music and sings about are very similar to the concepts that I personally believe and shape my life and coaching around.

One of my most favorite things about music is that it is a time machine! I absolutely LOVE how a song can take me back to a time and place. Whether it is memories from 35 years ago or just last week, music has a way of bending time! Think about it. In an instant you are back to a specific time and place!

When I hear songs from Fleetwood Mac, Boney M, ABBA and the Village People it takes me back to the 70's, when I was a young girl living in Winnipeg. I instantly have memories of our cottage, (oh, so many amazing memories of the cottage) playing sports and even the first time I went roller skating!

My decade of being a teenager began in the early '80's', the decade of one hit wonders. Many songs stand out for me. "Don't You Forget About Me" was my grade 9 Grad song. (I was awarded athlete of the year that evening. That was a great moment.) Every school dance was laced with Madonna, Michael Jackson, and Duran Duran. Anything Queen reminds me of watching the Live Aid concert back in 1985.

I remember my Mom always telling me how horrible the music was that I listened to. (I'm pretty sure her Mom told her the same thing). She would get her records out and say, "Now this is music." I listened for a minute, looked at her like she was nuts and said "I'm sorry Mom, but Slim Whitman isn't for me."

I find it amazing how when I am back in those moments they are as real as today. How awesome is it to flashback to a time and a place and relive some of those moments? Now, I am not saying that all of my memories are sunshine and roses. There are a lot of moments that I wouldn't want to revisit, even if I was paid. Thankfully, there is something called a skip, volume, or off button.

Music is therapeutic on so many different levels. I encourage you to pull out the music that moves you. Listen to it, sing to it, dance to it and create to it. Let music take you back in time. Let music help you dream about all the possibilities of your future. Let music create energy and build new memories today. Make music a conscious part of your life and enjoy the journey it takes you on.

Activity: Create a playlist for yourself that inspires you! As you grow and evolve, so will your playlist. You'll likely want to create several different playlists—those that calm and comfort you, one to inspire you, one that makes you feel playful or nostalgic, another to help you work out stress and adrenaline, and maybe one that piques your creativity… Whatever moods, feelings and mindsets you want to express, explore or delve into, create a playlist for that!

Letter to Cancer

I witnessed the power of this exercise at the Alberta Ride to Conquer Cancer in 2017 when one of the riders read his "letter to cancer" as an inspiration to the other riders. It was so clear that this man unleashed all of his anger and fears about cancer to the cancer that changed his life, and then he emerged from the darkness, feeling very empowered.

I believe doing this can be therapeutic in so many ways. When you write your letter to cancer, say everything you need to say to those sly little cells that have decided to camp out in your body. Don't hold back, say what you are feeling and get that energy out! Often shifting a mindset requires you to actively purge your feelings of fear and hostility, so set it all free!

In fact, I would encourage you to write your letter before starting your first leg of the climb. At the very least, get it started. You can write as many letters to cancer as you need to, but get the first one underway as soon as possible to start the purge. You may find that as you journey up the mountain you will have additional things to say to that thieving monster.

Be Kind to Your Support Team

This is more of a reminder than anything. As you embark on this journey, you are going to be challenged emotionally, physically, mentally and spiritually and so will your loved ones. The people around you care about you and want to help you make it to the top successfully. When you find yourself in the darkness, it might be hard to remember that they too are scared and sitting in their own darkness.

Please make sure you take the time to acknowledge their efforts, even when you think you feel justified to go off on them, rest assured they don't deserve it. Remember, they are trying their best to support you.

If anything, going through cancer highlights the fact that life is indeed precious. Depending on what stage you have been diagnosed with, anything can happen at any time up on that mountain. I encourage you to take the time and let your loved ones know how you feel about them, right here and right now.

Journal Entry: In the Living Years

(written February 2010)

It was my parents' 50th anniversary on Friday, February 12, 2010. I decided to prepare a speech. Taking the opportunity to honor my parents on their special evening ended up being a moment in my life that I will forever cherish. Here is why-

Six weeks prior to the anniversary, mom had a dry cough that turned wet, and we were waiting for the MRI results to find out what was going on. I had a sick feeling in my stomach and knew in my heart that my mom's time on Earth was drawing to a close. The last thing I wanted to do was have a party and pretend that everything was normal. There was also the pressure of coming up with a speech. How was I to come up with a speech for their 50th anniversary, when I was feeling so lost and upset, knowing that I may soon be losing one of my best friends?

I knew that on some level my dad knew that his wife, my mom, was not well. Planning and making it to his 50th wedding anniversary party was what was getting him through. I knew in my heart that him being able to say, "I was married for 50 years," was going be an anchor for him in the many years to come. Who was I, to not support and be a part of this significant milestone?

I had a choice. I could stay scared and small, or I could seize the opportunity to pay tribute to the people who were always there for me. So, I made the decision to support my dad and ensure that the memory of his 50th wedding anniversary would be special.

As I was preparing my speech, I was overwhelmed by the plethora of memories I had of my mom and dad. I truly led a blessed life on many levels. I had amazing parents! It was hard to come up with "just" a few things to talk about. After a few drafts, I came up with the perfect words to share with my parents.

This was the speech I prepared for my parents' 50th wedding anniversary:

"To have and to hold, for better or for worse, for richer, for poorer, in sickness and in health, to love and to cherish; from this day forward until death do us part."

Barrie and Norma went from being individuals, became a couple and then took on the role as parents. Today, as we celebrate their 50 years together, I get the opportunity to thank them for being great parents. As I reflect back on my life, words such as provider, teacher and friend, accurately describe some of the roles they took on when they became mom and dad.

As providers, they made sure that we were happy, cared for and loved. One such opportunity was to experience growing up carefree at our summer cottage in the Whiteshell. One fond memory is my dad getting up and taking me fishing at the crack of dawn. I ended up reeling in a fish twice as big as his. He says that he threw his two back because we didn't need that many. (I may have been young but it was pretty obvious why he threw his back). An example of providing us with a safe home, is coming home from school running in the front door yelling, "Hi mom," and always getting a response. We always knew that mom would be there waiting for us. We saw and felt support throughout all of our years of playing sports. Driving us to, from and all over so that we could play our sports. We could always count on one or both of our parents being in the stands cheering us on. I remember playing soccer in my teens, sometimes my mom was the only parent in the stands.

Mom and dad have been teaching us life skills as long as I can remember. Mom taught me how to get dressed (tag goes in the back) and how to make breakfast (bowl, spoon, milk). She taught me how to stand up for myself and "stick to my guns." She taught me how to embrace, in her words, "The independent little bugger that I am." Dad taught me how to tie my skates, ride my bike, how to cast a fishing lure and how to use tools. While mom gave us the unconditional "Mamma Bear Love", dad gave us the tougher "You can do it, I believe in you, love". My parents taught my brother and me, morals and values that gave us the foundation and structure to successfully build our lives to where they are today.

Their role as friends has always been there, but I know I only started to appreciate it over the past 20 years. Interestingly enough, that was just after I moved out. When I say friend, I am saying someone whom I can rely on, who is always there and is willing to help out in any way possible. As friends, they listen, encourage, accept and believe in me. When I call them, they always take an interest in what I say. Their unconditional love has always been there and is something that I will always cherish.

Barrie and Norma have ridden the many ups, downs and tight turns of marriage. They are currently experiencing one of the most challenging I do's of marriage, and that is the "For better or for worse, in sickness and in health" vow. Mom was once a vital source of strength for our family and her decline in health has brought forth a new strength in dad. Where once a woman led and looked after her husband and kids, a man has now risen, stepped up and is owning the responsibilities of that husband who said, "I do

They have touched many lives as individuals and over the last 50 years have influenced many lives as a couple. Everyone gathered here today to celebrate with them has felt their generous Spirit. Barrie and Norma have reached an incredible milestone in their journey together. They deserve to be acknowledged for the hard work and commitment they made to each other and their family over the last 50 years. While things haven't always been sunshine and roses, they found a way to make things work. I am proud to have you as parents and will always appreciate the people who you are.

I gave my speech and sounded like Mickey Mouse on helium as I choked out the words. My mom was focused on what I was saying. Her mind was confused, but I know in her heart, she felt the words I was expressing. My dad to this day, smiles and thanks me for what I "did for him and mom". I know the words I shared will always be in his heart.

Standing up in front of a group and being able to acknowledge and proclaim my adoration for the two people who made a life together, and raised me, was one of the best, most meaningful things I have ever done. Was it hard? Emotionally, yes. Knowing that I was saying thank you and good-bye to my mom was THE most difficult thing I have ever done. Was it rewarding? Yes. I feel very free on many levels. I will never have to wonder or have thoughts such as, "I hope they knew how much I loved them." "I never told them how great they were." "They were my parents I'm sure they knew."

We often think and assume that the special people in our lives know how we feel. Then, after they are gone, the guilt, constant worry and the wondering, "If they really knew," can eat us alive. Why live with unnecessary pain and anguish?

I am so fortunate that I made the decision to do that speech for their anniversary. If I hadn't, my mom would never had heard those words, and I would have been left wondering.

(My mom passed away 4 days after their 50th wedding anniversary. My dad passed away 16 months after their 50th wedding anniversary.)

Know with absolute certainty that your loved one knows how you feel. Do it NOW. Tell your loved one(s) how you feel while they are in their "living years".

CHAPTER 13:

Ready to Climb the Pink Mountain

As your pre-climb preparation comes to an end, I want to encourage you to fully immerse yourself in applying what you have learned and not just nod your head in agreement to the ideas and concepts. Just nodding in agreement means you have your head and heart in alignment, which is great. However, true transformation means acting on what you have learned. It is having your head, heart and feet in alignment! It means that with dedicated practice, you will become an expert on challenging your belief system, shifting your perspective and moving yourself out of a state of suffering and into a state of empowerment.

Throughout this climb and beyond, you will be placed in many situations that will cause Ego to go "bat shit crazy," and having the awareness to choose a Warrior Mindset and shut that fear down, will make a fundamental difference to your life.

Here is a personal example of this awareness in action. This was an update I sent out to family and friends six months after my treatment ended.

Journal Entry: Six Month Check-Up
October 2016

I had my six-month CT scan done last week and had follow up yesterday. I learned that I am good to go for another six months...Phew!

What exactly does that mean?

There are some "things" they want to follow up with in my lungs. I could interpret this news and live the next six months in one of the two ways. I could live in fear and conjure up a dark story in my mind about the Dr. being worried that the cancer has spread. Or, I could live from a place of power and know that the Dr. is doing his job, and my job is to continue getting strong and live my life fully.

When it comes to this cancer journey and climb, I listen to Blaze, my Spirit, and come from a place of power the majority of the time. But I do have moments when my Ego, Shade, manages to take control and feed me fear based stories. How do I know when Shade is up to her tricks? When I catch myself in a quiet, dark mood or I become quick to lose patience and I take my frustrations out on those around me. (That is usually on my partner Cheryl). I have come to notice, that my thoughts and actions preceding my Jekyll and Hyde moments are usually when I have spent time wondering about some of the crazy new symptoms that I have developed over the past three months, since I finished my cancer treatments. I truly believe that some of my symptoms are just my body recovering from chemo and radiation, while others are from Tamoxifen. However, every now and then, Shade slips in some shadows of doubt that cause my mind to go down the cancer rabbit hole, thinking that my symptoms are because the cancer has spread.

Here is how Blaze and Shade interpret my symptoms:

Blaze:

Headaches are from my hormones being completely out of whack from Tamoxifen.

Fatigue is from chemo and radiation.

Nausea is from my hormones being whacked from Tamoxifen.

Poor memory retention is from chemo and Tamoxifen.

Confusion is from chemo and Tamoxifen.

Blurred and weak vision over the last couple of months in my left eye is from chemo and aging.

All of my symptoms will go away with proper nutrition, exercise and time.

Shade:

Headaches could be from hormones, but it could be from brain mets.

Fatigue could be from chemo and radiation, but it could be from brain mets.

Nausea could be from my whacked hormones, but it could be from brain mets.

Confusion could be from chemo and Tamoxifen, but it could be from brain mets.

Blurred and weak vision could still be from chemo and regular aging eyes, but it could also be brain mets.

The reason why your symptoms aren't going away with your proper nutrition and exercise is because it is literally in your head! "Brain Mets!"

As you can see, Blaze and Shade have quite a tug of war going on about how to interpret this cancer thing of mine. To keep empowered and on Blaze's side of the rope, I engage in rituals that strengthen the bond to my Spirit. I read something positive and uplifting for 20 minutes every morning. I meditate for 20-30 minutes, followed by 30-40 minutes of exercise. This 1-2 hours of Cindy time, sets the energy and tone for my day and helps keep my feet firmly planted when Shade's fear based stories try to take me for a ride.

Finding 1-2 hours of "me" time is a challenge, that is why I get up early enough to do it first thing in the morning. I know for myself "later" never happens because too many things come up and all of a sudden I'm crawling into bed and the day is over. I also find that first thing in the morning, I am more open to receiving and creating that wonderful, positive, spiritual energy that helps kick start the day.

The time you spend meditating and connecting with your Spirit is quality time that literally "soothes your soul." The best part is you don't need any fancy equipment, shoes, clothes or space. You can do it anytime, anywhere, and all you need is the ability to close your eyes and breathe. (The only prerequisite for that is a heartbeat. If you are reading this that means you do have a heartbeat, so you are good to go!).

When I begin my meditation, I like to focus on the air flow as I inhale and exhale. I like to elongate my inhale to 4 seconds and then match my exhale with a 4 second count. As I do this, I feel my chest and rib cage expand and contract with each breath. As I settle into a comfortable rhythm, I state what I am grateful for. As I sink deeper into peace and calm, I go through my personal affirmations. I have mine typed out on a page that I read each morning. (I admit, I keep them in a plastic cover in the bathroom. Where else do you get uninterrupted reading time first thing in the morning?) When I am meditating, I say and mentally picture the words to my affirmations, which I believe help "turn the volume" up on the energy and vibrations that I am consciously putting out to the universe to support me.

I find spending 20 minutes reading material that opens and expands my thinking, helps to calibrate my energy and tone for the day. I then finish up my morning ritual with some exercise and stretching. By the time I finish showering, I feel a strong connection with my soul and my Spirit is soaring. I feel empowered when I start the day off standing on Blaze's side of the rope.

The days where I don't make time for my morning ritual, seem to be flat and dull. I am still productive and get things done, but I don't feel connected to what I am doing. When I don't feel connected, I seem to be quick to anger, or feel down and blue. This negative shift happens because I am tuned in to the whispers of my Ego. Shade absolutely loves it when I don't spend time fine tuning the clear guiding words of Blaze in the morning. It means the airwaves are open and Shade now has influence. Of course, I can course correct and fine tune anytime I want to throughout the day. The trick is consciously catching myself when I am playing out the drama that Shade is whispering to me. If I, all of a sudden realize, I don't like the energy I'm bringing to the situation, that is my cue that I am not tuned in to my Spirit. Chances are I am operating in automatic pilot with fear making the decisions, instead of being in the moment with love guiding me.

It's like listening to a radio station for hours and then you realize you are not quite tuned into the channel. You don't hear how distorted the sound is until you fine tune and hear the beautiful, clear music the "sweet spot" of the station's frequency brings. What you were listening to was fine, you could hear the songs and it got you through the day. But once you experienced the difference in sound when you fine tuned into the station, you realized there were two ways you could listen to your music. It can be good with some distortion, or it can be extraordinary with beautiful sound. Chances are you will choose to take the time to "fine tune" and listen to the extraordinary, beautiful sound.

If you want your soul to learn, grow and create to its full capacity, it needs to be tuned into the wisdom of your Spirit, Blaze.

Once experience the clear sound of Spirit, you will choose more and more to fine tune the station, when you realize you are listening to the distorted sound of your Ego. In other words, when you find yourself stressed, angry or depressed, you have the power to shift your perspective and move out of that distortion.

It is time to thrive your climb!

PART II:
The Climb

INTRO:

Thriving the Front Face of the Mountain

On any challenging hike that I have ever done, I would instinctively scan the terrain and break the climb down into smaller sections so I wouldn't get overwhelmed or discouraged by the vastness of what was in front of me. At the end of each section, I would stop, look at the beauty that surrounded me and acknowledge myself for completing it. When I made it to the top, I would proudly stand on what felt like the top of the world, do a 360-degree turn and truly take in all the moment had to offer.

It wasn't until many years later that I recognized that the feelings which were surging through me at the top of the mountains were feelings of love and gratitude. I was grateful for everything that brought me to the mountain, that got me up the mountain, and for the moment of grace at the top, as I connected with a power and energy that was so much bigger than me. The fortitude and lessons that I learned on those hikes followed me throughout my life. Anytime I faced adversity or challenges, I always took it one step at a time, kept my feet moving and tried to find the lesson and silver lining. I decided that going through breast cancer was no different. I pictured conquering cancer like hiking a mountain, and I would scale it with that same attitude, strength and fortitude that got me to the top of every other mountain.

Part II of this book is about getting you up the front face of the Pink Mountain, taking one step at a time, and applying everything you have learned in the pre-climb prep. You know how to shift your perspective and tune in to the whispers of your Spirit. You have the personal power to be in control of your thoughts, words and actions, allowing you to make conscious decisions that will create the results that you want. Remember, you can't control or change the event, but you can choose how you want to respond to it. You can either show up with a Victim Mindset or a Warrior Mindset!

Like all my challenging climbs, I broke the front face of this Pink Mountain down into five legs based on my experience with breast cancer treatment. By doing this, it allows you to stay focused on what is right in front of you, without getting overwhelmed with what lies ahead.

The Pink Mountain

(Legs of the climb)

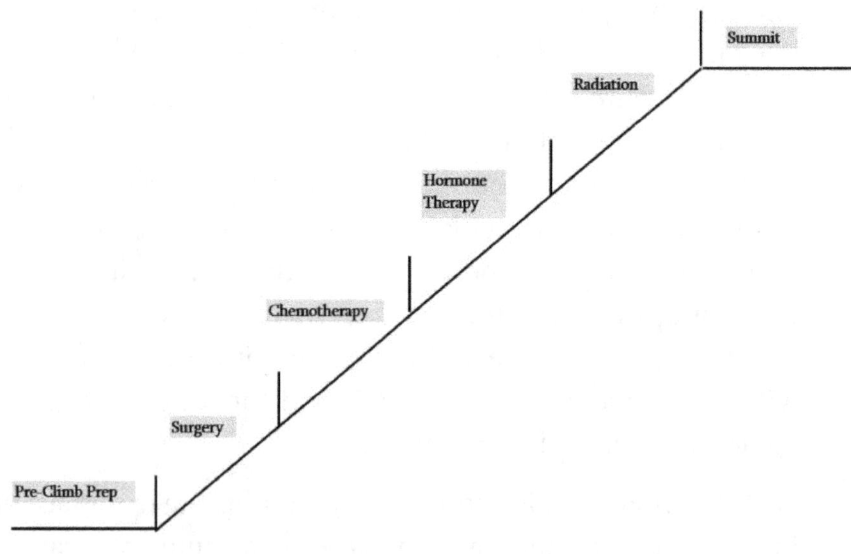

I start each chapter off engaging you with Big Picture Processing Questions. These questions will help kick-start the Rise Up process and your awareness into the Soul Games. With practice, you will begin to shift your perspective easier and faster each time you confront a challenge. Trust and follow the process and steps laid out here, and you will rediscover and embrace your inner warrior so you can thrive through your cancer journey.

Intro to: Big Picture Processing Questions

What two words describe how I feel right now?

• Asking yourself this question gets you to slow down, take a breath and determine how you are currently feeling. It helps you determine if you are sitting in a place of love or fear.

What is the worst-case scenario? What will my life look like if I have to travel down this road?

What is the best-case scenario? What will my life look like if I have to travel down this road?

• This is where you really need to visualize and understand both sides of the coin. This is where you become grounded in the bigger picture. By dismantling the fear, you will be able to keep a clear, more calm mind and begin to ask questions that will equip you on your journey up the mountain. Regardless of hearing either the worst or best-case news, if you aren't prepared, you will get lost in the emotion and shock.

Here is an analogy to help you understand why it's so important to be prepared with the best and worst-case scenarios.

Picture yourself watching an emotional movie for the first time. One of the scenes catches you off guard and you become a complete wreck. In fact, you are so absorbed in what just happened, that you tune out the next 10 minutes of the movie being worried and feeling lost in the scene you just saw. Eventually you regain your senses and continue watching. As the movie progresses, you are completely confused as to what's going on. The ending didn't make any sense and you feel angry about the whole experience. Afterwards, you reflect back on the movie and you realize you missed key pieces when you tuned out. Now you have to watch it again!

This time, you are prepared for the upcoming emotional scenes and they don't hit you as hard this second time through. Having an understanding of the scene, you have dismantled the shock and fear so you can focus on what is occurring now and what happens next. By the time the movie ends, everything makes perfect sense. You leave the movie feeling like you had a complete experience instead of a confusing mess.

Like the movie experience, if you run through the possible outcomes in your mind, discuss them with your loved ones (they need to prepare too), you will extinguish some of the shock 'now' so you aren't completely blindsided later.

Who do I want to be in relation to what I am experiencing here and now?

• This question allows you to be aware and consciously choose the mindset you want to show up with. It is always YOUR CHOICE!

What am I grateful for?

• Being grateful is accepting what is and being thankful for all that it is.

• Even in your darkest moments, there is always something to be grateful for.

For the record, because I didn't actually journal my BPP at the time I was going through cancer treatment, as I was just doing it instinctively, for the sake of demonstration I have answered them in each chapter of this book by going back and visualizing the moment and writing down what I felt was true at the time.

Speaking of going back, whenever I go back and read my journaling, I am amazed at how well I got through breast cancer treatment. I really do believe this is because I stayed connected to my Spirit. In my darkest moments, I managed to shift my perspective and move from fear to love. While coming from a place of love didn't change the journey itself, what it did do, was let me experience it from a state of empowerment.

I decided to include my journaling as examples of what climbing from a state of empowerment can look like. As you journey up this front face, I hope you find inspiration from my story, as well as learning to see and embrace that your experience of breast cancer is just more pieces of your soul's puzzle.

It is time to climb. YOU are a WARRIOR!

Tips and Tricks

Aside from my journal entries, I will also be sharing experiences that only if you're going through treatment will you really understand. I wasn't going to share these stories because I didn't want my experience to get in the way of your experience. I didn't want to add any more fear to your journey than you were already facing. Then, I got to thinking and decided that if you happen to face those same nasty side-effects, then maybe you won't feel quite alone if you knew what I endured. It's a highly personal journey, but in some ways, we are all in this together—you're NOT ALONE.

I also created this simple Tips and Tricks list to help a friend whose mom was going through breast cancer. I decided to include it here to help you plan ahead and be prepared in case those ugly side-effects come knocking on your door. Cheryl was at the drug store sometimes every day for the first week after my first round of chemo. Sometimes even twice in one day! By the end of the first month, I joked with Cheryl that she and the pharmacist were now on each other's Christmas card list.

Appointments

You want to make sure someone is at all appointments with you. Have that person making notes. This is not just for emotional support (it is that, too), but it's critical in making sure you are receiving all of the information you're getting. As much as you think you will remember everything, you won't. Knowledge is power. Don't be afraid to google reputable and legitimate sites to learn more about this disease and what it is you are facing.

Constipation

It's not **if** you get constipated by the steroid drugs administered before and after chemo days along with other medications, but **when**. I learned to be proactive with it by using over-the-counter medications that my doctor recommended. It's not fun, and it can be frustrating for that week, but it's so important to keep things moving, literally.

Water

It's very important to stay hydrated. I found room temperature water best. I started drinking 2 liters of water a day when I started chemo. I still do this. I bought a refillable, 1-liter glass bottle that I filled twice per day, and that way I knew I was getting at least two liters of water in. The glass is easy to clean. Not drinking enough water makes EVERYTHING worse, and it's a relatively simple solution when your digestive tract retaliates with vomiting and diarrhea. No matter what, keep track of your fluid intake, and keep drinking!

Food

Taste and smell will be altered and usually not in pleasing ways. Literally, it starts hours after chemo. The foods and beverages you love may now be completely icky. You will have a very heightened sense of taste and smell. Just roll with it. You will find things that work. It's important to make sure you are taking in high calorie foods, too. This is not the time to worry about taking weight off; that will likely happen on its own, and often quite rapidly.

At my worst times, I could only eat Ben and Jerry's vanilla ice cream (even Haagen-Dazs tasted wrong) plus Weight Watchers Banana Cream pie made with high fat Greek yogurt. (Sorry Weight Watchers!). You'll find what works best for you, but please do find something. It can be too easy to give up and just not eat—please don't do that! You need calories for energy.

Indigestion

My oncologist recommended Zantac and Pepcid AC. Have the conversation with your medical team to see if it's right for you.

Heartburn

This hit me hard three days after my first round of chemo. If I wasn't fit and healthy, I would have sworn I was having a heart attack. It was so bad that I threw up. I couldn't eat anything from the pain and discomfort. The oncologist gave me a prescription, and that got me back on track. It is a pill you take every day. I ended up taking it for five months. You will know when your GI tract is healed and you're ready to go off it.

Rest

I was so very happy just lying in bed in the dark with my eyes closed. I found too much noise and stimulation, whether it was good or otherwise, would overwhelm me, and I would start to feel sick and shut down. I liked being in the bedroom, but I could still hear conversation in the other room, so I still felt in the loop. Communicate with your loved ones so that they understand what you prefer and what works best for you—often people make assumptions because they care, and they are trying to think about what they would want if they were in your position. However, they are not you, they are not in your position, and they don't know unless you tell them. So, speak up, and be very clear.

Movement

When you can, get out and move your body! I managed to get out almost every day to the dog park. I was slow, but getting out is so important. Do the best you can. For peace of mind consult with your oncology team to get the go ahead.

Feeding your Soul

Keep your faith. As you are learning, your Soul has a purpose and your job is to keep picking up and placing the pieces of the puzzle together in your life. I really enjoyed my adult coloring book. It helped get me through some long nights. It was nice doing something creative that didn't overtax me. The better I felt, the more I could use my brain, but even if I felt awful, a simple activity helped me feel sane.

CHAPTER 1:

Surgery — Leg One of the Climb

Big Picture Processing Questions

- What two words describe how I feel right now?

- What is the worst-case scenario? What will my life look like if I have to travel down this road?

- What is the best-case scenario? What will my life look like if I have to travel down this road?

- Who do I want to be in relation to what I am experiencing here and now?

- What am I grateful for?

Even when you are prepared, you may still get some curve balls thrown at you. When you have done your research and have a better understanding of the bigger picture, you are able to ask more detailed questions when those curve balls happen. Being confident with who you are, and what your life will look like from those different angles, will help you remain calm and make sound decisions from a place of love instead of fear. Does this mean you won't feel the fear? No, your fear is real, but remember the swing analogy: You will go back and forth between Shade and Blaze. You have the personal power to dismantle your fear by being in control of your thoughts, your words and your actions. You are choosing to come from a Warrior Mindset. You are dialed into your Spirit and making conscious decisions, instead of being pulled around by the fear of Ego.

Before surgery, I had a consultation with the surgeon to decide the best course of action to handle my tumor. I went in prepared, with a little knowledge on all the different stages of breast cancer, so I could have a bird's-eye-view of the bigger picture. In saying this, I focused most of my research on stages I and II, as well as the ins and outs of a lumpectomy and mastectomy as treatment protocol. From where I was standing, the best-case scenario would be a lumpectomy, worst-case scenario a mastectomy. My biggest fear that Shade kept creeping in with was, "OMG, I don't want to have a uni-boob!"

When my mind took off like that, I just gently reminded myself that I would cross that bridge when and if I got to it, and if that was the best course of treatment, I'm sure they have technology to balance the girls out.

I answered these BPP questions based on how I remember feeling when I was preparing to see the surgeon.

What two words describe how I feel right now? I am a strong, fit, healthy, vibrant woman.

What is the worst-case scenario? That a lumpectomy would not be enough, that I would need a mastectomy, or perhaps a double mastectomy. **What will my life look like if I have to travel down this road?** I could be a uni-boob. I imagine there are procedures that will balance out my chest back to "normal". It will be painful a process, but I am strong and will make it through. If it's both breasts, what will that look like? Well, I know I am more than just my breasts. We had a 32 year run, but if they are trying to kill me, it's time for them to go.

What is the best-case scenario? A lumpectomy! **What will my life look like if I have to travel down this road?** Normal. It will change nothing. I will experience some pain, but overall it will be a speedy recovery.

Who do I want to be in relation to what I am experiencing here and now? I choose to be fearless. I can't control the situation, I can only control how I choose to respond. No matter what the outcome, I know I will be ok.

What am I grateful for? For living in a province that has incredible support for women going through breast cancer. I am also grateful for my partner Cheryl.

So how did things go with my appointment? Here is the Boob Update from my journaling:

Journal Entry: Boob Update
September 23, 2015

Hi Guys,

So I met with the surgeon today and this is where we are at. (BTW, once you are in the system, things start to move and shake)

I learned I have two things going on:

1. I have a mass that has been diagnosed as invasive ductal carcinoma (IDC).

2. I have a large segmental cluster away from the mass that is highly suspect of ductal carcinoma insitu (DCIS).

The recommendation is a mastectomy because with both issues going on, to get clean margins (to get all cancer cells), they will have to take too much breast tissue as a lumpectomy.

Because of genetics, and not wanting it to come back in the other breast, I will be getting a double mastectomy.

I will be contacted in the next two days with a surgical date.

During this surgery, they will be taking out the first 2-3 lymph nodes in my left armpit and sending those to pathology as well. This is a standard procedure to see if any cancer cells are present in the lymph.

Once the pathology is examined, they stage the cancer.

Stage I-is localized in the breast.

Stage II-means they found cancer cells in the lymph.

I'm keeping my fingers crossed for stage 1!

2-4 weeks after surgery, if needed, I will be seeing an oncologist.

I am still confident that things have been caught early and I will come out on top! It may be a bit of an ugly climb, but I am still going to kick it's ass!

Big hugs and love, Cindy

I want to be clear. Having a Warrior Mindset does not mean stuffing your fears. It is important to feel whatever it is you are feeling. A Warrior Mindset means that you have the conscious ability to recognize where on the swing you are sitting. You have the power to shift your perspective when sitting in the darkness no longer works for you. I will be saying this a lot throughout this book. You don't know who you are, until you experience who you are not. I remember coming out of appointments and Cheryl would ask how I was doing. Sometimes, I told her that I just needed to sit in the darkness for a moment. I needed to understand where I was at and how I was feeling. I reassured her that I would be fine, that I just needed to process it all.

I would like to point out that your people, your support team, might also need to sit in the darkness as they too are processing things. That is why it is important to keep the lines of communication open on both sides, as this journey impacts everyone. Everyone involved needs to feel what they are feeling. Your loved ones may feel embarrassed talking about their fears to you, because they aren't the ones going through cancer and that they need to be strong for you.

I remember driving home from the appointment with the surgeon and Cheryl was in a bit of shock, still trying to catch up to the fact that I was getting a double mastectomy. I was feeling calm because I had been preparing myself for all outcomes. I knew that no matter what, I would be fine. Cheryl on the other hand was still trying to put the pieces together. I remember telling her, "It's ok sweetie, we will get you through my double mastectomy." She looked at me and started laughing and said, "How bad is it, that you have to get me through your double mastectomy?" That was when I really recognized the importance of both, the patient and the support person, talking through their fears. She didn't stay in the shadows for long, just long enough for her to take a bird's-eye-view and see the bigger picture.

Once Cheryl caught up, we were good the rest of the climb. If at any time Cheryl felt bad for thinking she was letting me down, I would say, "Don't worry sweetie, we will get you through my double mastectomy," and then we would just laugh.

In fact, part way through my climb I noticed, whether I was talking to someone or reading my journal, I always said, "we" when referring to the major steps of the climb. That was because Cheryl was very much with me every step that she could. I knew where she was at, and she knew where I was at, because we kept the lines of communication open.

Pre-Surgery

Pre-Surgery Big Picture Processing Questions

Please take a moment to ask yourself these Big Picture Processing questions.

- **What two words describe how I feel right now?**

- **What is the worst-case scenario? What will my life look like if I have to travel down this road?**

- **What is the best-case scenario? What will my life look like if I have to travel down this road?**

- **Who do I want to be in relation to what I am experiencing here and now?**

- **What am I grateful for?**

The morning of surgery I was actually quite calm. I attribute that to my spiritual practice and grounding. I had done some additional research about mastectomy and sentinel nodes once I got my actual surgery date. Having that understanding of how those two major parts of my surgery connected, took any apprehension away. Here is my grounding the morning of surgery.

What two words describe how I feel right now? Nervous, faith.

What is the worst-case scenario? That my surgery gets botched and I am completely deformed. That they find the cancer has spread past what they thought. **What will my life look like if I have to travel down this road?** I will have some body image issues that I will have to work through. Hopefully, there is a procedure that could fix it. If the cancer is more extensive than originally thought, then I will decide the best course of treatment for me and my life.

What is the best-case scenario? That the surgery goes well, the cancer is contained, and I heal up like a champ. **What will my life look like if I have to travel down this road?** I am a healthy woman and with my education and background in fitness and wellness, I will get back on my feet in no time.

Who do I want to be in relations to what I am experiencing here and now? I, Cindy, am here to be the "Big Me". I am whole and complete. My body is a gift to experience my life with.

What am I grateful for? That I am catching this early and I have a lot of living to do.

Doing BPP can also help you keep your cool when you are just coming out of anesthesia and your nurse isn't quite familiar with your file yet! Let me share this story with you.

I was coming out of the anesthesia in the hallway as I was getting wheeled into my room. Just like in the movies, shaking off anesthetic is a bit of a process.

As I was regaining my senses, a nurse came buzzing in and while she was taking my vitals, was asking me the usual questions. Can you tell me your name? Do you know what day is it? Do you know what procedure you had? I answered with confidence, as I did the 10 times they asked before surgery. The only difference this time when I answered, a double mastectomy with a left sentinel node dissection, the nurse blurted out, "No. You had a left mastectomy and a partial right mastectomy." Then she buzzed out of the room as fast as she came in. I was left lying there, somewhat stunned and still doped up, thinking, "OMG! How did this happen? They got it all wrong. Hurry up and wheel me back down so they can fix it!"

I reminded myself to take a deep breath and trust my faith that my surgeon did what he was supposed to. I needed Cheryl there so she could get to the bottom of things, but she wasn't there yet. That was when another nurse came in. As she got closer to me, I recognized that it was my friend, and nursing student, Alison. I was so happy to see Alison! She would straighten things out! I told her my situation, her eyes got big and she left. I wasn't sure if that was a good thing or a bad thing. I trust my friends to have my back, so I knew Ali would help.

After what seemed like forever, the original nurse came running back in, apologizing that she gave me the wrong information, and that I did indeed have a double mastectomy with a left sentinel node dissection. For the record, that was a long and confusing few minutes!

Moments later, Alison came back in and asked if I was ok, and then she did the simplest thing. She gently raised the neckline of my gown and took a peek. Yes, they were indeed both gone! I have to say, I never even thought of doing that. That would have saved me five minutes of unnecessary stress!

The nurse came in and apologized again and thanked me for being so calm. I was thinking "Calm? I didn't feel calm!" In fact, I was panicking that my worst-case scenario came true! That's when I realized that my grounding and pre-climb prep did its job, which was to mentally prepare me for any curveball. Even though I felt panicked, I was still able to stay calm and rational in a high stress moment.

Post-Surgery

Post-Surgery Big Picture Processing Questions

Being that this was a major surgery, they kept me overnight in the hospital. It was when I was by myself that I started to think, "Wow, this really happened. This is really happening! I have breast cancer and I just had a double mastectomy." Before the imagination of Shade could take off, I took a few deep breaths and contemplated my grounding questions.

What two words describe how I feel right now? I am a strong, fit, healthy, vibrant woman!

What is the worst-case scenario? That I get an infection or the cancer has metastasized. **What will my life look like if I have to travel down this road?** It will be a temporary setback, but I will get through. If it has metastasized then I will cross that bridge when I get there.

What is the best-case scenario? Everything went as planned. **What will my life look like if I have to travel down this road?** I believe my breast cancer was caught early and I am going to live a long, healthy life.

Who do I want to be in relation to what I am experiencing here and now? As the reality keeps sinking in that I have said good- bye to the girls, and that I have breast cancer, it's important that I keep my faith throughout the process. I know that this is part of my soul's journey and I will continue to do my best to understand the greater purpose as it presents itself.

What am I grateful for? My health and for Cheryl's love and support.

If, after your surgical procedure, you catch yourself starting to panic or lose control, remember to ground yourself. Write in your journal, feel what you are feeling and then decide who you want to be in relation to the moment that is presenting itself to you.

Remember, every moment of every day is an opportunity for you to experientially know who you are in relationship to this world. Like a single snowflake that is unique in design, so is your soul's journey.

Journal Entry: Post-Surgery Update
October 20, 2015

Good afternoon,

Seeing there are no more boobs to talk about, it is now just "the update".

I have made it home, safe and sound and I would guess, about 6 or 7 pounds lighter.

My surgeon did an amazing job and I can't say enough positive things about him. A great surgeon like him both medically and professionally, sure makes this whole process easier. I feel pretty blessed that he was my Dr for such a "delicate" procedure. He said my incisions have excellent lines and should heal very neat and tight.

The Dr. decided to take a 4th lymph node while he was in there. Anything that looks "suspect" is easier to take out and send to pathology now, rather than having to go in a second time. Better to be over cautious than not!

I have 3 drains that will stay in for 10-14 days. Cheryl, me and home care will be looking after those. The nurses assured us that they are easy to maintain. (They are more a nuisance than anything.) Home care will be coming in every 2 days to help with drains, bandages etc..

My follow-up is booked for November 5th and that is when we will learn the stage of this cancer and what the course of treatment will be. So, for now, it is all about the rest and recovery for both Cheryl and me.

Thank you all again for your love and support throughout this process. It has been very heart felt and is making this journey that much easier.

Home Recovery

Big Picture Processing Questions

Please take a moment to ask yourself your Big Picture Processing questions.

- **What two words describe how I feel right now?**

- **What is the worst-case scenario? What will my life look like if I have to travel down this road?**

- **What is the best-case scenario? What will my life look like if I have to travel down this road?**

- **Who do I want to be in relation to what I am experiencing here and now?**

- **What am I grateful for?**

Getting home can be scary for both you and your caregiver. Between the pain, drugs and learning a new routine, you may find a shortness in patience. On the first night home, Cheryl and I were watching tv and all of a sudden, I needed to go to bed, not now, but right now.

I managed to get my teeth brushed and then we needed to empty my drains. That's when things got testy between us. Cheryl was afraid of pulling too hard on my drain tubes and them coming out, so her milking effect seemed to take forever and was not very effective. We weren't sure of anything and a lot of choice words were being mumbled. We did the best we could considering all of the newness and uncertainty. We were both tired and exhausted, and it showed.

This was just the first leg of the pink mountain. I knew we would have a long journey ahead and Cheryl, as my caregiver, would need her sleep. Ultimately, I ended up sleeping in the spare room, as I was in pain and very restless.

As I lay there awake, I had time to reflect on our milking the drains episode. It will be a long six months, if that was an indication of how we handle the hurdles ahead. I meditated, shifted my perspective and did my BPP.

What two words describe how I feel right now? I, Cindy, am a loving, caring, and compassionate woman.

What is the worst-case scenario? If I continue to react in frustration to Cheryl trying to help me, we will end up resenting each other. **What will my life look like if I have to travel down this road?** This will be a very long and lonely road.

What is the best-case scenario? I take the lessons from my shifted perspective and recognize that, in the event of another heated moment, I need to pause for the cause, take a deep breath and choose to respond in a proactive way. **What will my life look like if I have to travel down this road?** Much happier! Both Cheryl and I will feel loved and appreciated.

Who do I want to be in relation to what I am experiencing here and now? I want to be aware and respectful of Cheryl and her efforts helping me on this climb.

What am I grateful for? Cheryl

That next morning Cheryl came upstairs and we decided to empty the drains with me lying down. Each drain had its own measuring lines and once we milked the lines using some hand cream on our fingers, we were good to go. By the second draining that night, we were full on pros! It also helped that when the home care nurse came by that afternoon, she showed us that there was no worry of the drain tubes coming out, as they were a good 6 to 8 inches inside of me.

Speaking of the home care nurse, we knew that my bandages would be coming off and that we would be seeing things for the first time. By this time my grounding questions were becoming automatic. (You will notice I often use more than two words to describe my feelings.)

What two words describe how I feel right now? I, Cindy, am a beautiful, confident, powerful loving woman.

What is the worst-case scenario? The bandages come off and I look like the bride of Frankenstein. **What will my life look like if I have to travel down this road?** I will be looking at additional surgeries down the road to repair things.

What is the best-case scenario? That I continue to feel whole and complete. **What will my life look like if I have to travel down this road?** Continue to feel acceptance and love for who I am and be at complete peace with my new body without breasts.

Who do I want to be in relation to what I am experiencing here and now? I am and always will be, a beautiful, confident, powerful loving woman.

What am I grateful for? That my personal development work has brought me to a place where I can process myself and be in a state of acceptance instead of blame and anger.

Journal Entry: Coming Home Update
October 25, 2015

Good morning,

Well, what a week! I have to say this had been an interesting ride so far.

I came home Tuesday with three drains. Two of them were on my left side (which is called the affected side and where I also had lymph taken out) and the third is on the right side. It is up to Cheryl and me to monitor, empty and record the fluid coming out of each drain. Our first evening home was a bit of a gong show, but we now have this process down to a science.

Once a drain records less than 30 ml over the course of 48 hours it is allowed to come out. Last Friday, one of the drains on my left side came out, so I am now down to just the two.

The home care nurse comes to the house every second day to check things out and calls every day for updates. If we have any issues, they would come out to the house immediately. Both Cheryl and I feel confident in the system and have no worries.

We saw things for the first-time last Wednesday when the nurse changed my bandages. Cheryl was watching the bandages come off and didn't even blink an eye. All I saw was love and compassion in her eyes. I took a look and saw how great of a job my surgeon did.

Cheryl and I have had many conversations and some laughs about my new look. One of the funniest is how Cheryl is now the "endowed" one in the family. The other bizarre but funny thing is, when I am sitting with my shirt open and everyone is taking a peek, it doesn't feel like I am exposing myself. There is nothing to expose!

I did amazingly well the first few days, I had pain but it seemed pretty mild, but then all of a sudden on Friday, it was like everything woke up and it woke up angry. I have about 5 different kinds of pain that constantly light up at different times. I am very thankful for pain medication!

The other thing I am very thankful for is the TEAM of support I have around me.

When Cheryl and I came home on Tuesday, our "Kentwood family"(our wonderful neighborhood friends) let us know that they would be bringing us dinner every night. We also had friends and Cheryl's family drop off some soup. This was one of those things you don't really understand the impact of until you experience it. The look of relief in Cheryl's eyes each night when one of our neighbors dropped off a meal filled my heart with love and gratitude. You see, looking after my needs, the dogs and her own needs has been a full-time job for Cheryl. Not having to worry about feeding us in this first week of adjustment, has been a tremendous weight off Cheryl's back. I can't express enough of how this gesture made that much of a difference to our week.

Emails, messages, cards, gifts, and flowers that I have received help feed my strength and keep a smile on my face. Thank you all for that.

Finally, I just want to take a moment to thank Cheryl. I would not be recovering like I am without her. Cheryl has given me 360-degrees of love and support. She had a stressful spring/summer dealing with an aging parent, computer glitches with her business, her own nerve pain from her back surgery last summer, and then learning of my diagnosis in August. These last five months have not been easy for Cheryl, yet this week, probably our hardest week, she has found a way to rise up and be my rock. Even though we have never said the words "in sickness and in health" to each other, there is not a moment that goes by where I don't feel that love, devotion, and commitment from Cheryl. I am truly blessed.

Thank you all for your continued love and support.

Staging Results

Big Picture Processing Questions

Please take a moment to ask yourself your Big Picture Processing questions.

- **What two words describe how I feel right now?**

- **What is the worst-case scenario? What will my life look like if I have to travel down this road?**

- **What is the best-case scenario? What will my life look like if I have to travel down this road?**

- **Who do I want to be in relation to what I am experiencing here and now?**

- **What am I grateful for?**

As I was recovering from surgery, I understood that I could have either stage I, stage II, or depending on lymph node involvement, even a stage III diagnosis. This is the first time I began to even entertain the idea of stage III. I began preparing myself for my appointment with the doctor by getting a clear understanding of what each stage meant, the treatment plans related to them, and of course, the prognosis. I also did my grounding around my current understanding of all three stages.

What two words describe how I feel right now? I, Cindy, am a strong, fit, healthy, vibrant woman.

What is the worst-case scenario? Being told I have stage III breast cancer. **What will my life look like if I have to travel down this road?** Treatment will be the same as stage II but the prognosis is different. I will be looking over my shoulder and most likely be always worried about the cancer coming back.

What is the best-case scenario? Being told I have stage I. After learning about stage III, this is truly the best diagnosis with the best prognosis. **What will my life look like if I have to travel down this road?** I will get back to what my life was like before cancer more seamlessly.

Who do I want to be in relation to what I am experiencing here and now? I am a true warrior and I can handle whatever diagnosis news I am handed.

What am I grateful for? My body and the miracle that it is.

Journal Entry: Staging Results
November 4, 2015

Good afternoon,

Well, I just have to say, for the record, that a double mastectomy is a brutal process! The first 2 weeks after surgery were pretty rough. (I won't go into detail, as it is now in the past.) On the plus side, I am starting to feel better and having significantly less pain. I hope to start some physiotherapy in the next week to get some mobility in my left chest/shoulder.

We saw the surgeon today and my incisions are looking good. He did drain some of the excess fluid. I guess it's quite common to get a fluid build-up. (I was starting to feel like I had me some girls again.)

My surgeon also gave us the results of my pathology. When it was all said and done, there were 7 lymph nodes that came out. They did find cancer in one of my lymph nodes, so I have Stage II Breast Cancer. What this means is I will be seeing an Oncologist and will be needing chemotherapy and possibly other adjuvant treatment, such as radiation.

On a positive note, the Surgeon made the right call on the mastectomy. The segmental cluster had a lot bigger surface area than originally thought and was classified as DCIS with a grade III, meaning- that, even though it was contained, it was aggressive and would have gotten ugly fast. To get clean margins between it and the actual tumor, I would have had no boob left anyway.

Even though this is a Stage II cancer, I believe

that it was caught early. I know that chemotherapy/radiation will take care of any other cells that may be lurking in other lymph nodes. It will also annihilate any stray cells that may have gotten past the nodes and are window shopping for a new home. I may be a good host, but only to the people I love. These cancer cells are going to get found, kicked out, and killed!

So, when does all this happen? Well, first I have to heal from my surgery and that is a six-week window. My referral to the Oncologist will be going in today. It may take up to 4 weeks to see him, which will be that magic six-week mark. If it takes a little longer to see him, it just won't matter, as the more healed I am, the better shape I will be in for radiation and chemo.

How am I doing with all of this? I am doing ok. I know things were caught early and I'm going to live a long, healthy life. I'm doing this once and only once! No surprises for this girl 2, 5, 7 or 10 years from now. I am kicking ass on this now! There isn't any mountain that I can't climb. I have my game face on and this journey will unfold how it's supposed to, and I am going to finish stronger than ever.

Thank you all for your continued love and support. It's way easier to climb this pink mountain with you on my team.

The doctors have a general idea what stage you are most likely at, by the size of the tumor, when it is originally found. This general idea helps them figure out the best order of YOUR cancer treatment plan. Remember, it is not a 'one size fits all' approach to treating breast cancer. There are so many factors that doctors look at to determine the best course of treatment. Some women like me had surgery, chemo, hormone therapy, then radiation. Where other women may have chemo first, then surgery, hormone therapy and radiation.

Regardless of your treatment order, it is a hard mountain to climb. You can't change your diagnosis, the only thing you can control are your thoughts, words and actions about it.

CHAPTER 2:

Chemotherapy—Leg Two of the Climb

Big Picture Processing Questions

Please take a moment to ask yourself your Big Picture Processing questions:

- What two words describe how I feel right now?

- What is the worst-case scenario? What will my life look like if I have to travel down this road?

- What is the best-case scenario? What will my life look like if I have to travel down this road?

- Who do I want to be in relation to what I am experiencing here and now?

- What am I grateful for?

In the couple of weeks in between my staging and actual oncologist appointment, I had some time to do research on chemotherapy, understand my current beliefs about breast cancer and do my big picture processing. I actually went through the Belief System Cycle in detail because I found myself anxious, and quite worried about the idea of chemo, which was causing me to lose sleep and become way too preoccupied about it. I felt that my agitated behavior needed some extra attention, so this is what I learned.

Belief System Cycle

(Please refer back to the Belief System Cycle chart on page 19)

Chemotherapy is a neutral event.

My belief system says: OMG, you are going to be so sick and bald! This was reinforced in my family groove by watching my parents' reactions when people, whom they knew went through it in the "old days".

Thoughts and feelings: Nervous and scared about putting poison in my body.

Words and actions: I said fuck a lot.

Results: My mind was running wild with fear, thinking of every movie I ever saw of people going through cancer, which reinforced my current belief system.

My Big Picture Processing questions specific to chemo helped me pause my thinking and "Rise Up". I was able to shift my perspective and move into the Soul Games.

What two words describe how I feel right now? I, Cindy, am a strong, fit, healthy, vibrant woman.

What is the worst-case scenario? I go bald, get sick and catch an infection. **What will my life look like if I have to travel down this road?** I need to be hospitalized and isolated, so I don't die from a serious infection.

What is the best-case scenario? That treatment is way different than it used to be and symptoms will be mild. **What will my life look like if I have to travel down this road?** Sure, I might be bald, but like the cancer treatment itself, it will soon pass.

Who do I want to be in relation to what I am experiencing here and now? I want to stand tall and continue staring fear in the eye.

What am I grateful for? My faith and meditation.

Looking at my "chemotherapy Belief System Cycle" after meditation and Big Picture Processing.

Chemotherapy is a neutral event.

My Belief system says: This is all just temporary.

Thoughts and feelings: I know everything happens for a reason. This is just part of my journey.

Words and actions: I am a strong, healthy woman and I will get through this.

Results: While I am nervous about the chemotherapy, I want to make sure I do everything that will kill this cancer.

My blog post after my sit-down with the Oncologist.

Journal Entry:
Next Steps Chemotherapy
November 25, 2015

Good afternoon,

It's been 5 weeks since my surgery and I am doing better every day! As long as I am falling forward, I am happy.

I met with the Oncologist yesterday and learned what my next steps are going to be. For the record, Dr. W. is a beautiful human being and I have full confidence in him and the treatment plan he has put together.

I will be undergoing four hits of chemotherapy and maybe radiation. (We will learn more about that once chemo is done and I see the radiation oncologist). I will also be having a ten-year relationship with the hormone drug Tamoxifen. Apparently ten years is now the magic number to get to, before a person is considered cancer free.

Below is how I understand the how's and why's of my breast cancer as well as how next steps will work:

All cells have receptor sites (basically antenna), that collect hormones so they can grow and do their job. Every receptor is shaped for a specific hormone so other hormones can't accidentally get picked up (think lock and key). In the breast, when cells need to grow, the ovaries call for more estrogen and progesterone to get picked up at that site (breast). The cell sends out a specific number of receptor sites that collect just the amount it needs. Most of the time this happens flawlessly. If communication lines do get crossed, our bodies are very intelligent and have a defense system that is fantastic at hunting down and destroying cells that try to mutate and start problems.

Now, in the case of a "genetic" mutation, the cell has figured out how to disguise itself until it can grow to the point where it has built up an army. Once this army is built up (tumor), it then likes to break out and set up shop in other areas of the body such as organs (metastasize). Once it sets up new camps throughout the body, the chances of controlling the rogue cells become less and less. This is why early detection is the key to survival.

My genetic mutation posed as a breast cell and put up extra "estrogen" receptors (antenna) to disguise itself and grow. Because of this clever "genetic involvement", my defense cells didn't pick up on its radical behavior. My cancer is ER+, (estrogen receptor positive) which means it likes estrogen. It is also Stage II, which again means cancer cells were found in my lymph, which means it has broken out with the intention of setting up new camps.

The best plan of attack, to hunt down and kill any rogue cells window shopping for a new home, is chemotherapy. One of the many side effects of chemo is that it will depress my ovaries, so the call for estrogen will slow/stop. When the chemo ends, we will start hormone therapy with the drug Tamoxifen. This has a dual effect. One, it will put me into instant menopause (so again, no more estrogen) and two, because Tamoxifen molecules are shaped to fit the estrogen receptor sites, if a rogue cell is in hiding and tries to call in estrogen, Tamoxifen shows up instead. It will no longer have an estrogen source to grow with.

Over the next couple of weeks, I will be getting a couple of baseline tests done. (This gives us a peek at what my organs look like now, so over the years if there are any changes, they can hone-in-on them). Instead of mammograms, I will be getting scans.

As far as when I will be starting these next big steps, we have been given the option to start in January after our trip to Mexico, (that we had booked/paid for back in July, before this gong show began). The Dr. says I am just on the edge of the magic window (evidence shows a greater success rate in the first 3 months after surgery). Because I am flirting with the edge and not going past it, the Dr. is ok with my taking this time and feels it will be of benefit in my recovery process. We have a couple of days to decide.

If we go, that means I have an extra month to recover from the mastectomy (which is good because my range of motion is only at 70%), strengthen my body (get cardio and stamina up for the effects of chemo), and have a mental break in the sun with Cheryl before going into this next body-altering step. AND I will still have hair for Christmas!

My job and focus are to look after my mind, body and Spirit, so I come out the other end of this journey healthy and strong. While I am not happy about the idea of chemo and instant menopause, I am happy to know that over the years, research has evolved and treatment has become specialized instead of a one size fits all. I believe that going through another 5-7 months of ugly is a drop in the bucket compared to the many years of life I still have left to live.

Thank you for your continued love and support.

Sitting with the oncologist and learning the in's, out's and why's behind my type of breast cancer and understanding the prognosis from all angles, helped to reinforce that I was making the right decision for me. As much as I was not happy about bathing my body in chemicals, I felt more confident in doing it because treatment is more targeted now. It is not just a blanket approach like I had learned and stored up in my Book of Life from my Family Groove.

I think that it is important for you to research, ask questions and feel confident in your decision to go forward or not with chemotherapy. As always, the decisions are in your hands, that is why you want to make sure you are participating in that decision-making process.

Here is what I ended up doing…

Journal Entry: My Final Decision
November 26, 2015

Good afternoon,

The last 24 hours of decision making are over.

I woke up this morning, feeling quite confident thinking that I had come to a decision about when to start chemo treatment.

I felt that having the extra time to recover from surgery would be highly beneficial. It would also give me the time to make a game plan to keep as healthy as I can during treatment. (Apparently, the anti-nausea pills really work, but it may really stimulate appetite causing weight gain.) I wanted to make sure I had a solid eating plan in place where I could monitor what I was eating and make sure I had a balanced food portfolio.

I also felt that taking time to reconnect with Cheryl in Mexico would help us recover from these last few months and get us ready for the next 5-7 months.

I was getting ready to call the Dr. with my decision when I got a funny feeling in my stomach. I decided to Google 'time between surgery and chemo'. I began to read some sobering studies and their outcomes.

Studies show optimal success rates getting treatment in the first 30-60 days depending on stage of cancer.

with stage II cancer, going past that date range can change the survivor success rate.

I understand why Dr. W. was slow and hesitant in saying he would be "ok" with it. While an extra month of healing and time relaxing in the sun would benefit me, it "may" also change my survival stats. Ultimately, he left the decision up to me, but I really would be flirting with a razor's edge.

I just had a huge "A-ha!" moment writing this. I've been looking at this from only one angle. We only get one shot at life and we should take opportunities and seize them. On the surface, that opportunity is honoring my "fun side" and going to Mexico. But really, the opportunity being offered to me is the chance to get treatment immediately and live a long, healthy life with many trips to Mexico.

My head and heart have aligned and I am making a clear, "soul" decision. I am choosing to seize my life, Mexico can wait. I finally feel at ease and very empowered with this decision.

I will be bald for Christmas!

Thank you all for being with me on this up and down decision. Time to call the Dr. and get this process started!

As you can see, being dialed in to the whispers of your Spirit, will lead you to the decision that sits right with who you are. Reflecting back, I am so glad I made the decision to go ahead with treatment and postpone Mexico. One of my philosophies throughout my cancer treatment was to go big or go home and leave no stone unturned. I didn't want to have a recurrence down the road and beat myself up thinking, "If only I did this. Or if only I did that."

You will start to notice as you pay attention and apply the Rise Up process, that your ability to tune into your Spirit becomes faster and quite natural.

Chemo Round One

Big Picture Processing Questions

Please take a moment to ask yourself these Big Picture Processing questions.

- **What two words describe how I feel right now?**

- **What is the worst-case scenario? What will my life look like if I have to travel down this road?**

- **What is the best-case scenario? What will my life look like if I have to travel down this road?**

- **Who do I want to be in relation to what I am experiencing here and now?**

- **What am I grateful for?**

I know that there are many different kinds of chemotherapy and depending on what type of breast cancer you have, you will most likely have a different response than I did. In fact, two people with the exact same chemo will respond somewhat differently. They may have similar and predictable patterns, but ultimately, their bodies will process things slightly differently. My experience may not turn out to be your experience, but the reason I am sharing my journaling is because it demonstrates the importance of staying with your Warrior Mindset. Remember, you can't control that you have breast cancer, all you can control is how you respond to it.

I learned quickly into my chemotherapy treatment that I was facing a fierce battle physically, mentally, emotionally and spiritually. As I felt myself wanting to give up to the dark side, I did my BPP (Big Picture Processing)

Here is my blog after my first round of chemo:

Journal Entry: The Battle
December 13, 2015

Good afternoon,

It took me a few days, but I was finally able to string some words together...

Chemotherapy is rough. Very rough.

Even with adequate warning, I was still blindsided by the harsh effects of chemotherapy.

The first few days, I was caught off guard by waves of pain that left me feeling pretty defeated. My body hurt in so many different ways, I lost count. (It still hurts.)

Even the ability to enjoy some of the simple pleasures in life, like coffee and chocolate, has become impaired. Coffee has taken on a less than pleasant soapy taste and chocolate feels like it's burning my tongue.

while a tongue that feels three inches thick, and a body that feels like it's on fire, can make it difficult to rest, it was the numbness creeping into my mind, body and spirit that started to get my attention.

I found myself wanting to tune out everyone and everything. I caught myself thinking, "Whatever happens will happen. I'm not in control anymore. Whatever". In the middle of my sad story, I decided that sitting in the darkness and being a victim to the battle going on inside of me certainly was an option, but not my option. I decided to honor my spiritual warrior instead.

Here is what my spiritual warrior knows, I do have control. The mind, body, Spirit is a very powerful connection and when they are out of balance, I have the choice to put them back together again. Instead of being a victim to the battle inside of me and just accepting whatever might happen, I am choosing to visualize a battle of good vs evil. I am choosing to be connected to this battle with all of my being.

With every wave of pain that hits me, I know that to mean that the cancer cells are being hunted down and killed off. Pain and discomfort does not defeat me in this battle, it is just an indicator that I am winning this war!

This is what I know to be true:

I, Cindy, am a strong, fit, healthy, vibrant woman.

I, Cindy, am here to be the BIG Me!

Thank you for your love and support as I dig deeper.

First Round Side Effects

I found that doing "normal" though out the chemo treatments was important. I got down to the dog park most days. It was funny because I thought I was walking fast and ripping up the trails. Three quarters around the park Cheryl finally asks if we could walk a little faster as she was freezing. I didn't realize it, but we were walking so slowly, she was almost walking backwards! So, I guess even if you think you are doing normal things normally, you might be doing just a slightly different speed and version of it. That's fine, by the way!

I also tried to maintain my fitness routine the best I could. My game plan was to do what I could when I could. I had a sneaking suspicion that my "best" would change as my cancer treatment compounded, and I was extraordinarily correct.

The thing that surprised me the most was how much my senses got altered, though. My sense of taste and smell became so acute that to this day I still can't stand certain foods or scents, which prior to treatment I enjoyed. Three hours after my first chemo I couldn't eat or stand the smell of bread because of the very intense yeast-smell it "suddenly" had. I remember having a bite of chocolate, and it felt like my tongue was burning. Then, the next morning I had a sip of coffee and couldn't figure out why it was so soapy. I thought that perhaps the carafe wasn't properly rinsed. When Cheryl tried it, she said it was fine. Later that day, I popped a piece of gum in my mouth, and I couldn't spit it out fast enough. It tasted like a mouthful of chemicals. I can see why people lose weight through this process. Finding something that my sense of smell and taste could stomach was a challenge! However, going through the process of discovering palatable foods is critical to your health!

Two weeks after that initial Chemo, I tried a glass of my favorite wine at Christmas. I got the glass a few inches from my face, and all I could smell was chemicals. Instead of complaining about my altered senses, I decided that it was a gift. Clearly, whatever is in these foods and beverages I had so fondly enjoyed, they're not necessarily healthy for me. Just because over the years I acquired a taste for them, doesn't mean I should be consuming it.

For the record, three years later, I still can't stand the smell or taste of flavored coffee, gum, or Zinfandel and Shiraz wine. It is sad but true!

The worst thing I experienced after the first round of chemo was not the hair loss; that actually didn't bother me too much. More on that in a bit... The worst thing, other than the yeast infection, occurred on the fourth day. Halfway through the day, I was struggling to get a full breath. It felt like I had something stuck in my chest. When I went to lay down, I had such an intense pain behind my breast-bone, I was beside myself in pain. If I wasn't in such good shape, I would have sworn I was having a heart attack. As it turned out I had extreme heart burn from the chemo stripping my esophagus cells. Since it was the weekend, I managed the best I could with over the counter antacids. The only position I was comfortable in was standing. That first night I was in agony, so I stood at the kitchen island and distracted myself by coloring in my adult coloring books. (By the way, these were great for keeping my mind preoccupied throughout my cancer treatment. I got to be creative without too much thinking.) Eventually Monday came, and thankfully I was able to get some serious medication to assist with heartburn for the duration of my treatment. They worked like magic!

When I sat down with the oncologist, he mentioned that at the two-week mark I would lose my hair. So, two weeks before chemo I prepared for the hair loss by going extra short on my haircut. It was short enough that I was annoyed whenever I saw my reflection (I figured bald would probably actually look better than what I was currently sporting). I never gave much thought to losing my hair, because I was distracted by other issues such heart burn, constipation and yeast infection. Then, one morning as I was putting goop in my hair, I suddenly had more hair on my hands than Chewbacca!

I was stunned for a moment and ran to the calendar. It was December 23. Yup, I was one day shy of that two-week mark. Dang! The doctor was bang-on with that side effect! By the next morning, my hair was coming out in chunks. I messaged my neighbor and beautiful friend Tanya and asked if she would be willing to shave my head. She told me to come by after lunch that day.

That same morning, our friend Peggy came by and surprised me with a merino wool toque. I told her she had good timing, as my head was getting shaved after lunch Now, here is a perfect example of why communication with your loved one is important. Cheryl pivoted around and said "What! Today? Maybe you can wait until after Christmas!

I had been preparing for the hair loss the moment I learned I would need chemo. I had done my BPP and was quite fine with it all. I wanted it shaved. Not just to say goodbye to my bad hair style, but so I could quit watching it fall out in chunks.

I told Cheryl to hold a chunk of my hair. I turned my head and she was left standing there holding a mass of my hair. She looked shocked and then said, "Okay, I just need a minute to catch up."

I thought we were on the same page about shaving my head when my hair started to come out. As it turns out, Cheryl knew I would lose my hair, but she hadn't done any kind of BPP to truly ground herself in what it all meant, so it really did take a moment for her to catch up to the reality of it all.

Hair Loss

I would recommend doing BPP around hair loss. This is what mine looked like.

Big Picture Processing Questions

Here is what my BPP looked like around hair loss.

What two words describe how I feel right now? Calm and in control

What is the worst-case scenario? For some freaky reason my hair doesn't grow back! **What will my life look like if I have to travel down this road?** I would rock my bald head or commit to a wig.

What is the best-case scenario? That I look good with a bald head and I will finally heal the dry patch I've had on my scalp for the last few years. **What will my life look like if I have to travel down this road?** It is only hair. It will grow back.

Who do I want to be in relation to what I am experiencing here and now? Confident. I will appreciate any kind of hairstyle, whether it be a good one or a botched one. I know that like my breasts, my hair does not define who I am.

What am I grateful for? Having a wonderful partner who loves me and for having an incredible and caring friend, who wanted to help ease my transitioning to bald in the chill of an **Alberta** winter.

Once Cheryl and I talked through both of our feelings, she was quite fine. She did just need a few minutes to catch up to where I was already standing. After lunch we walked over to Tanya's and had some laughs as we shaved my head.

Chemo Round Two

Big Picture Processing Questions

Please take a moment to ask yourself these Big Picture Processing questions.

- **What two words describe how I feel right now?**

- **What is the worst-case scenario? What will my life look like if I have to travel down this road?**

- **What is the best-case scenario? What will my life look like if I have to travel down this road?**

- **Who do I want to be in relation to what I am experiencing here and now?**

- **What am I grateful for?**

It was at this point in my journaling and updates, when I realized that I was getting through those first few legs of cancer treatment (and the gong show that went with it) with a strong mental fortitude because I was dialed into my Spirit. I was consciously shifting my mindset through meditation, affirmation and grounding myself.

Remember, meditation isn't always about sitting on a cushion repeating mantras. Through some of my darkest and most trying moments, all I did was close my eyes, focus on my breathing, and repeat my personal affirmations. Doing this always seemed to calm my body, mind and Spirit. When I felt that sense of peace wash over me, I would shift my perspective to see the bigger picture. After I analyzed both sides of the coin, I would feel grateful and at one with my Spirit.

With Big Picture Processing, I created a simple way for you to get to that "oneness" with your Spirit. A Warrior Mindset doesn't just happen, it takes awareness and dedication. The more consciously you do your BPP, especially in those moments that you are feeling somewhat defeated, you will feel a shift in your mindset and you will feel the power of Blaze. The more empowered you become, the more faith and fortitude you will build to carry you through those seemingly impossible events.

I skipped right to my blog post(s) because it basically encapsulates my BPP in the raw.

Journal Entry: Chemo II
January 7, 2016

I've been asked, how is it that I am able to keep my spirits up going through all of this cancer/chemo.

I pondered that question, because it's true, I have been enduring some really hard moments both physically and mentally through this journey so far. Most recently, the chemotherapy has definitely had its share of punches.

Aside from the normal, ugly, side effects, during the first chemo, I developed a rash on day 7, that caused me some unpleasant issues for a couple of days. I was told that it was a reaction to the chemo drug and that for the second round they would reduce the dose. I felt that it was an allergy reaction to the Neulasta, (that gets injected subcutaneously the day after chemo), which is a drug that boosts the immune system by helping the body increase its white blood cells. The doctors and nurses insisted that they have never seen an allergy to it, and they were confident that it was the chemo drug.

So round two of chemo happened, with a reduced dose of the drug they felt to be the issue, followed with an injection of Neulasta as scheduled the next day. Two hours after the Neulasta shot, I developed a head to toe, rash and hives. The doctor and nurse asked me to come back to the hospital immediately so they could evaluate me. After their jaw dropping reactions to seeing first hand, my hot, raised, blister like skin, my health care team agreed, that I do indeed have an allergy to Neulasta. For them, I was the first "allergy" case they have ever seen! For me, it meant enduring 5 days of an allergy, that came and went 6 times a day, in unpredictable patterns, creating intense skin pain, shortness of breath and exhaustion.

As I write this, I am amazed that I finished going through that ugly experience only 3 days ago. It feels a lot longer than that! The human body is nothing short of a miracle. Just three days ago, my body was a complete war zone! It was responding to a severe allergy, while managing the cell stripping, energy zapping chemo drug...AND, my already taxed out system even graciously responded to the additional assault of Benadryl and prednisone for 5 days!

Every day, I learn something new about this incredible vehicle that houses our soul, and I continue to be blown away by the gift that it is.

So, how do I keep my spirits high? It's because I have absolute faith and knowingness that I am a strong, fit, healthy, vibrant woman. This is just a part of my journey and will be over soon enough and I will be stronger for it. I also know that every moment of every day, I get to choose how I want to view the events in my life. I can choose to be angry at the world and at my body for putting me through this, or I can choose to thank my body for being so amazingly resilient, while I am ridding myself of cancer, so I can enjoy a long, healthy life.

Even in the middle of that ugliness, I was thanking my body for being so strong. (Albeit, a little scared, curled up in the fetal position, buried in blankets, focused on just breathing and feeling my heartbeat, in a dark, quiet room for hours on end, while Cheryl looked on worried and feeling helpless.)

For the record...Regular chemo side effects will seem a little easier to handle after experiencing that allergy. At least they are predictable, familiar, somewhat short-term, and manageable.

Journal Entry: Lucky Numbers 12 and 7
January 11, 2016

Number 12 and 7 are now two of my favorite numbers. Let me share with you the reason why.

A week ago, I was on the tail end of a five-day allergic reaction to an immune boosting drug. Today, 12 days after my second round of chemotherapy, I woke up feeling more rested, clear headed, and light in Spirit. While I am still experiencing chemo side effects, such as compounding fatigue, and the "surprise of the day" location where the chemo is playing, day 12 seems to be the day I feel a shift. I feel my body coming back into balance spiritually, emotionally and physically.

I noticed this positive shift in balance on day 12, after my first round of chemo. If patterns prevail, this means that these next 7 days are my "power" days. Like cresting a hill on a bike, I am going to enjoy the feel of the downhill ride, rest my body, and gain momentum before heading up the next hill.

Like on my last series of power days, I will focus on what makes Cindy strong. I will eat nutritious food to boost my immune system, ride my bike or elliptical trainer to keep my heart strong, and continue to do my stretches to keep my back, legs and fresh incision scars from getting stiff.

Here is a little confession. On my first round, I didn't realize I was going to get seven power days. I remember waking up after 11 very rough days thinking, "Hmmmm... I feel good today. I have some energy, my taste buds are back and I have an appetite. It's Christmas...I am going to eat whatever I want." It was an absolutely wonderful day, and I enjoyed every moment! To my pleasant surprise, I woke up each morning for a week with the same feelings and enthusiasm to indulge in all the yummy baking that surrounded me. (Thank you family, friends and neighbors for making those seven days delicious!)

Now, I can't stay healthy and keep my girlie figure doing that each round of chemo. I have maintained a healthy, strong, vibrant life because I honor a balanced lifestyle. When I first learned of my diagnosis and understood the toll it would take on my body, I promised myself that I would do everything in my power to help keep that balance. I know having a strong heart and body can make a world of difference in how I heal and how quickly I bounce back from surgery and then chemo. Aside from Christmas week, I have done a really good job at consistently moving and stretching (minus the really ugly allergy days).

My level of health and fitness is nowhere near it was before all of this started. My best varies day to day, and that's ok. I keep my head in the game, and the strength I do maintain, will carry me up the discomfort of the next hill, to the light of another day-12 and the body recharge of seven power days.

I love the numbers 12 and 7!

Thank you for being a continued source of love and support. Your emails and kind, positive words help keep my spirits high.

Chemo Round Three

Big Picture Processing Questions

Please take a moment to ask yourself these Big Picture Processing questions.

- **What two words describe how I feel right now?**

- **What is the worst-case scenario? What will my life look like if I have to travel down this road?**

- **What is the best-case scenario? What will my life look like if I have to travel down this road?**

- **Who do I want to be in relation to what I am experiencing here and now?**

- **What am I grateful for?**

Here is my BPP before going into the meeting with the oncologist to discuss round three.

What two words describe how I feel right now? Determined and anxious

What is the worst-case scenario? What will my life look like if I have to travel down this road? I could go into anaphylactic shock. I may have permanent, cellular damage that will negatively impact my life.

What is the best-case scenario? What will my life look like if I have to travel down this road? The doctor agrees with me, we go back to full strength chemo. My body will recover from the chemo like the millions of people before me.

Who do I want to be in relation to what I am experiencing here and now? I am in tune with my body and I want to help it get through this experience in the best possible way I can.

What am I grateful for? Knowing myself and my body well enough that I know when to fight hard and not back down.

Here is my journaling for round three:

Journal Entry: Allergy or Not

January 14, 2016

Good afternoon,

Here is a quick update after meeting with Dr. K. (oncologist) to discuss next week's chemo plan.

Both he and Dr. W (my lead oncologist in Calgary), still believe that it was the chemo drug Dosetaxyl that is causing the allergy. I strongly believe it to be the Neulasta (immune boosting drug) that is the culprit, and I refuse to put it in my body again.

Keeping all of this in mind, the new plan for round 3 next week is as follows:

i) We are going to go ahead with the chemo drug but, because they feel it is the culprit, they want me to take Benadryl prophylactically, starting the day before chemo and continue for 5 days. I am to have a script ready for Prednisone, if I develop an allergy like last time.

ii) Without the Neulasta to boost my white blood cells and platelets, I am to be super diligent the first 10-12 days about having or getting any kind of infection, cold or flu. I am to have a script ready for antibiotics at the first hint of anything.

Now here is the interesting part.

i) If I don't have an allergic reaction on number three, I am golden. I can finish off with chemo number four with the same Dosetaxyl drug.

ii) If I develop an allergy equal to or worse than last time, they won't be able to administer the fourth round of chemo with Dosetaxyl.

What this means is they will put me on a different chemo drug, and here is the sucky part, I will need extra rounds of chemo! (Boo)

Bottom line, next week when I have my third chemo treatment, we want NO allergic reaction. If I do get an allergy reaction, I will have to change drugs and face extra rounds of chemo.

So please pray for me to be allergy free! (We also want to stay healthy and not catch any, infection, cold, flu, fever or virus because that would be bad.)

Journal Entry: Spotted or Not
January 30, 2016

Good morning!

I am very excited to announce that I have no spots! (I am doing a happy dance).

The doctors said I needed to be allergy free in the first 10 days before they could rule out the Dosetaxyl (chemo drug) as the culprit. Well, here I am on day 10 with no allergic reaction! I knew that if I made it through the first 24 hours I would be golden, but I also know that anything can happen with chemotherapy, so I waited until this decisive day 10 to update you.

No allergy means it was the Neulasta injection (as my body highly suspected), which means I can continue on with this Dosetaxyl and finish my last chemo treatment as scheduled on Feb 10. YAY!

As far as any additional side effects, I do feel more tired and fatigued than last round. It could be because my red blood counts are wiped from not taking the Neulasta, or it could be the compounding effects of the chemo. Overall though, I think I am doing FANTASTIC!

Journal Entry: Next Step Radiation

We met the Radiologist this past week to discuss whether I need radiation or not. In my head, I was thinking that the double mastectomy, chemo and Tamoxifen was going to be enough to slay the cancer beast, so I was really hoping to hear the words, "You don't need radiation." Alas! No such luck for this girl. Bottom line, studies and research indicate that once cancer cells make an appearance in your lymph nodes, they take on a whole new level of deception and evil. The best counter attack is to bring out the big guns at every turn to make sure all angles are covered.

Ultimately, treatment at every step is my decision. Throughout this whole process, Cheryl and I have listened to what the doctors had to say. We asked a lot of questions, (we have been told by the Drs., nurses and students, that we ask a lot of excellent questions) and then I make a decision on what I feel is best and true for me.

As much as I was hoping to not need radiation, I am in this to win! I am not going to fight and battle all the way down the field and then stop on the one yard line. I am charging through, into the end zone, and am taking this win away from that silly thing called Cancer!

When does this charge to the end zone start?

They give me a month to strengthen up from my last chemo session. So, in the last week of February, I get set up and measured for my radiation specific beam pattern, and then treatment begins March 14 and goes every day for three weeks plus a day.

Until then, I want to thank everyone for your love and prayers. Your positive thoughts have created a very powerful, healing energy for me throughout this journey.

I really do believe the human body is a miracle. Going through cancer treatment is sound proof, that it can take a licking and keep on ticking. (It's not super happy about the chemical bath, but at some level it knows how to get through). If you pay attention and listen to your body, you will begin to notice patterns like I did with my lucky 12 and 7.

The reason I encourage you to pay attention and get to know your body is, so you can be your own advocate, especially when you really feel something is not quite right. Using my allergy to Neulasta as an example. The doctors had never seen anyone with an allergy to it, so they thought it was the chemo drug. I absolutely felt, without a shadow of doubt, that it was the Neulasta. I went with them on their theory for round two, and things went sideways fast. For round three, I absolutely refused to put the Neulasta in my body. During round three, I'm pretty sure I heard my body sigh in relief.

If you have been in tune with your body over the years, paying attention to it throughout cancer treatment won't be too much of a stretch for you. If going through cancer treatment has awakened you to begin paying more attention to your body, that's fantastic.

Remember, you are a three in one being. You are Mind, Body and Spirit, and being aware of and maintaining balance between the essence of these three, will make your ride here on Earth way more fun.

I wrote this back in 2014 and think it talks to this point beautifully.

Journal Entry: Legs of Life
2014

Mind, Body and Spirit- our legs of life.

Like a three legged wood stool, when one of the legs is short or missing, the stool is not stable. To correct the problem is easy. Just trim the longer legs down. Ta da, problem solved! Yes, the problem is solved but only for a moment. If we keep cutting the legs back to match the short leg, our beautiful stool will eventually become nothing more than a wood disc, not at all the beautiful wood stool that we started with.

Like the three legged wood stool, when one of our legs is ignored, we are not stable.

Chances are, at any given time throughout our lives, we are living with a short leg and we feel out of balance. Just as we get one leg all balanced out, suddenly we are out of balance with another leg! It seems like we are always chopping our legs down. Soon, we won't have anything left. It's exhausting!

So how about adding length to our legs to balance out instead of cutting back the others?

To do this, you always need to be aware of all your legs.

Mind, Body and Spirit work together. When one is out of balance, the others bring strength to it. This takes awareness. To live life to its fullest you need a balance and understanding of your Mind, Body and Spirit.

What is a strong mind?

Understanding the difference between decisions driven by Ego or decisions driven by Spirit. There is no right or wrong. Based on the outcome of your decision, a strong mind driven by Spirit will either take a step back and course correct, or take a step back and reflect on what went right. An Ego driven mind will either say this didn't work because of all these reasons or say this worked because I am genius and better than everyone else. It was all me, me, me!

Being aware of how you are showing up is living consciously. We are here to learn and grow as we navigate the journey of life that we have been given. To navigate our journey we need a destination, a map, a compass and a vehicle.

The importance of a healthy body

If you are planning a trip somewhere, you will need a mode of transportation. It could be a bike, a car, plane, or boat. No matter what the mode, you want to make sure it is in good working order so you have a safe, comfortable, reliable trip and make it to your destination.

Our journey through life requires a mode of transportation and we have been given a miraculous vehicle to do just that. The human body is fully equipped to take us on our life's journey! Like a vehicle, if you properly maintain and fuel your body you will have a comfortable ride as you learn, grow and create through life.

Keeping your spiritual warrior present

(Being a spiritual warrior)

Living spiritually aware, is knowing who you are and what your purpose is. This can happen consciously or less than consciously. Living from Spirit, is those moments we have, where everything just seems to line up for us. It is that moment of greatness and aliveness that we feel in every fiber of our body. When it just happens, it is because our innate purpose and actions were in alignment. With dedicated practice, you can achieve these moments everyday. The volume or magnitude will change from moment to moment, but fulfilling your soul's purpose can be, and should be, a daily event.

Chemo Round Four

Big Picture Processing Questions

Please take a moment to ask yourself these Big Picture Processing questions.

- **What two words describe how I feel right now?**

- **What is the worst-case scenario? What will my life look like if I have to travel down this road?**

- **What is the best-case scenario? What will my life look like if I have to travel down this road?**

- **Who do I want to be in relation to what I am experiencing here and now?**

- **What am I grateful for?**

I skipped right to my journal post(s) because it encapsulates my BPP in the raw.

Journal Entry: Near the Top
February 15, 2016

I just finished my fourth and final chemo treatment. I am very happy to be done with this leg of the climb. I believe I was able to maintain a positive attitude during this "chemo climb" because I focused on one step at a time. Even during the turbulence of allergies and body rash, I kept my head in the game and focused on getting through each moment. All steps needed to be completed, to help build a strong foundation to keep pushing off from.

Throughout this cancer journey, I have made sure I had knowledge of the terrain. I spent time learning and educating myself on all possible angles, so I could adapt to any sudden changes. I felt that if I understood the hazards, I could do a better job at staying on track. I have also listened to my heart and soul, and have maintained a strong climbing body.

As with any mountain, the higher up you get, the more chance of a misstep. Fatigue sets in and focus becomes a little skewed. Fatigue may also weaken your fortitude enough for your mind to play fear games with you. Seeds of fear may start sprouting, telling you stories that may not even be true for you. For example, to keep you "safe", fear may tell you that being close to the top is the same as getting to the top. That those last few meters are the most dangerous, and perhaps the view is just as good from down lower. Fear isn't telling you this for its own well being, it's telling you this because fear is afraid of the 'unknown' that may be lurking up there.

Even though your initial goal was to scale the mountain, stand on top, and breathe in your victory of conquering such a feat, fear has managed to cause you to second guess yourself. Fear would rather keep you uncomfortably comfortable than risk stepping into the unknown and have to adapt, change and do things differently.

To continue to climb or not, needs to be an informed decision based on facts, an understanding of the terrain, experience, and a serious heart and soul check. Such a critical decision should not be left for fear to make. If we cave in to fear and turn around before the summit, without the opportunity to explore our options, we may live with the regret of never knowing our true potential and face a lifetime of second guessing that fateful decision.

I still have a couple of big pushes to complete before I hit the top of my cancer mountain. These last two treatments that were once at a distance away, are now just a step away, and they were starting to drive my fear factor.

It's only been in the last two days that I have been able to shift my perspective and really see things. I realized instead of me being in control, I was letting fear take the wheel. My head was so far ahead of "what is", that I was spinning in circles and getting dizzy. No one can make a clear decision when they are dizzy!

I know there are possible side effects to radiation, and I know that there will be unpleasant side effects to the hormone therapy that will create instant chaos throughout my body. (What hasn't thrown my body into instant chaos on this climb?) I also know the human body is intelligent, and if I choose to listen to it and honor its wisdom, I will be able to bring it back into balance and restore my vibrant energy. It may take a while, but I will bring it back into balance!

Instead of letting fear hold me back, I am choosing to push for the summit and finish this climb. I would rather stand at the top and put my body back together piece by piece, than let fear take away my heart and soul!

This Too Shall Pass, and through a dedicated practice......Time Will Heal All Wounds!

Journal Entry: Hitting the Milestones
March 2, 2016

Milestone One was getting through surgery.

As of today, I feel like I have officially finished Milestone Two, which is completing chemotherapy.

Here I am, three weeks after my last chemo, and I don't have to get ready for another round. Today feels pretty frickin' amazing! I am so relieved to be done with that poison.

I have to say, for the record, this final round of chemo has been a kicker. The side effects and events of the last five months have compounded. My body is fighting hard to regain its health and vitality. I keep reminding myself that rebuilding a body takes a lot of energy as cells work at replenishing themselves. I guess that is why babies only focus on sleeping, eating and pooping, as building a body is a lot of work. It seems at times that is all I have the capacity for.

Another interesting side effect that I started having two weeks ago is a phenomenon called "chemo brain." I never knew such a thing existed until I started having symptoms. I welcome you to Google "chemo brain" to get a full appreciation of this affliction. (Thankfully, Cheryl, going through menopause can relate to my momentary mental "gaps".) Between the two of us playing fill in the blanks, we can generally string together a pretty decent conversation.

Now I am preparing for the next big step...

Journal Entry: Radiation Set Up

I had my "set up" radiation appointment this past Monday. I learned more about the process, which gave me more confidence in the whole idea of receiving radiation treatment. It really is pretty amazing how pin-point accurate everything is, thanks to advanced technology. **Actual treatment starts March 14, and goes three weeks plus a day.**

All my measurements and images were done under a CT scan, so they are specific to my body and breathing pattern. These images will be sent to four different levels of medical doctors to be examined, templates made, and then cross checked before they are signed off on. (Picture an image you outline using tracing paper. The tracing paper image would be like my template, which all future treatments are lined up with).

I have been tattooed so the CT scanner, templates and radiation beams all line up and play nice! (The tattoos aren't as bad ass as they sound. It's just three markings across my rib cage. I have moles that are more bad ass!) During treatment, my live images, as seen under a CT scan, must line up with my template, or the radiation beams won't turn on. (This is a fail-safe switch, so I don't get accidentally nuked somewhere else). For example, if I suddenly move or cough, my live image would not be aligned with the template and the radiation beams shut off instantly.

Like I said early on in this journey...

Here is what my spiritual warrior knows... I do have control. The Mind, Body, Spirit is a very powerful connection and when they are out of balance, I have the choice to put them back together again. Instead of being a victim to the battle inside of me and just accepting whatever might happen, I am choosing to visualize a battle of good vs evil. I am choosing to be connected to this battle with all of my being. I am choosing to be a warrior!

With every wave of pain that hits me, I know that to mean the cancer cells are being hunted down and killed off. Pain and discomfort does not defeat me in this battle, it is just an indicator that I am winning this war!

This is what I know to be true:

I, Cindy, am a strong, fit, healthy, vibrant woman.

I, Cindy, am here to be the BIG Me!

It feels amazing to have these two massive milestones under my belt. As I take a moment to celebrate, I want to thank each and every one of you for your support along the way. Knowing, I have you cheering me on along the way, keeps my feet moving. We are almost at the top, my friends!

As I read back on these journal entries, I find myself simply amazed at the fortitude we as humans have, especially when we choose to honour our "Life Force" and choose a Warrior Mindset.

The compounding effects of the cancer treatment was noticeable. I kept thinking how blessed I was for being healthy and fit going into it. I can't say enough of the importance of doing your best to maintain good eating and some form of exercise. Every little bit does make a difference and thankfully there are local support groups to help you get on track if you need that extra encouragement.

I believe staying strong on all fronts was the reason why I was still able to make those hard decisions with confidence. It is so easy for you to bail on yourself and let others make those critical decisions for you, that way if something goes wrong, it's easier to blame someone.

"Chemo brain" is an interesting phenomenon. More on that at a later date. In the meantime, my best advice is for you to keep your sense of humor and not be so hard on yourself. Your body is trying to deal with a lot of things and something has to give, so if that happens to be certain aspects of your brain, just know that you are in good company with the rest of us climbers.

Chemo Brain

Big Picture Processing Questions

I would recommend doing your BPP around chemo brain. It will help you accept the process with a smile on your face. Here is what mine looked like.

What two words describe how I feel right now? Frustrated and tired

What is the worst-case scenario? That I never get my brain or energy back. **What will my life look like if I have to travel down this road?** I will have to accept what is and alter and change what I do in life. I may not be able to keep my current job.

What is the best-case scenario? That this is just super temporary and I will get back to normal in no time. **What will my life look like if I have to travel down this road?** Nothing will really change for me.

Who do I want to be in relation to what I am experiencing here and now? I am a warrior and I will never give up on myself.

What am I grateful for? I am grateful to have a supportive and loving partner who is willing to work with me as I adjust to these radical changes.

Cheryl was super supportive with my chemo brain. That could be because she had menopause brain and truly understood the brain gaps which I was experiencing. I would go into another room to get something and completely forget what I was doing. Cheryl could hear that I had stopped dead in my tracks and was paused. That's when I would hear a loving reminder of what it was that, I was doing.

CHAPTER 3:

Hormone Therapy—Leg Three of the Climb

Big Picture Processing Questions

Please take a moment to ask yourself these Big Picture Processing questions.

- **What two words describe how I feel right now?**

- **What is the worst-case scenario? What will my life look like if I have to travel down this road?**

- **What is the best-case scenario? What will my life look like if I have to travel down this road?**

- **Who do I want to be in relation to what I am experiencing here and now?**

- **What am I grateful for?**

I didn't journal the start of hormone therapy, but I do remember the moment clearly. I stood there holding the little Tamoxifen pill, knowing that as soon as I swallowed it, my body chemistry was going to blow up. I didn't know what to expect, I just knew that estrogen is a key hormone that I, as a woman, needed! When women go through menopause naturally and their ovaries shut down, the body still secretes a trickle of estrogen through the adrenal glands. So, artificially shutting down my estrogen supplies cold turkey did make me a little nervous.

I remember my BPP clearly,

What two words describe how I feel right now? Nervous and apprehensive

What is the worst-case scenario? If I don't take this drug, there is a high percent chance of my breast cancer coming back. **What will my life look like if I have to travel down this road?** I will be forever looking over my shoulder, scared that any little symptom of anything and nothing, would mean the cancer is back. I would be mad at myself for not doing everything at the time to give myself a shot at the best prognosis and future.

What is the best-case scenario? Is that my body sails through this easily. It is possible. There are some women that go through menopause without a hitch. Maybe even though I am artificially altering mine, I am still one of those women who will breeze through it! **What will my life look like if I have to travel down this road?** Nothing will change.

Who do I want to be in relation to what I am experiencing here and now? I am a warrior and I didn't come all this way to give up on myself now.

What am I grateful for? I am grateful that there is research and targeted therapy that give people going through cancer a fighting chance at life.

Going through chemically induced menopause has been a challenge, but I always remind myself of the alternative. Sometimes, I get a little angry, thinking I have been brain washed with this fear, but I know at some level, keeping my estrogen blocked is my best chance at survival.

*** It has been about six weeks since I wrote that last paragraph and I have the perfect story of how Tamoxifen has become such a part of my life that the idea of not having it caused panic.

My Story: Mexico Trip

The night before leaving for Mexico, I counted out and put together my medications for the trip. I remember picking up the blue blister pack card of Tamoxifen and danced down the hallway to the rhythm of my thyroid and 5HTP shaking in the bottle. I put them in my backpack instead of the suitcase to ensure that they made it safely to Mexico, if for whatever reason my suitcase didn't.

The next evening, as I was getting ready for bed, I went to set out my water, thyroid and Tamoxifen for the morning. I reached into my backpack and pulled out the bottle of Thyroid and 5HTP and as I reached back into the backpack my hand started moving around in a pure panic. I could not find my Tamoxifen! I frantically stripped through the whole backpack. Cheryl just as concerned, went through all of our toiletries, suitcase and backpack as well. It was nowhere! I recalled the night before when I was packing. I remembered looking at the blue card and I remember dancing down the hallway. That's when I began questioning myself. Perhaps, I picked the card up and then put it back in the drawer when I was putting together the Thyroid bottle? Maybe, I forgot to grab it when I began dancing to the rattle of the other meds? At any rate, I did not have it! I was in pure panic.

For the record, I wasn't concerned about the cancer coming back in ten days, I was quite scared at what my hormones were going to do! Vacation is not the time to go cold turkey on hormone suppressing drugs! I didn't know what the next 10 days would bring, but I knew it would be hormone, ping pong hell and that would not be good for me or anyone around me!

After going through several laps of my Belief System Cycle, that was loaded with F-bombs, I moved into the critical junction. I knew I couldn't change the situation. I could only choose my response, and in that moment, I shifted my perspective and accepted what was. It was 11:30 p.m., and there was literally nothing I could do at that time. I was tired from a long day of travel and decided I could make better decisions in the morning. I crawled into bed and had a good two hours of sleep before my mind started up again.

I woke up feeling agitated, and began beating myself up for being so careless with my Tamoxifen. I once again caught myself after a few laps around my Belief System Cycle, regained my Warrior Mindset and came up with a plan. It was a half-baked plan, but a plan nonetheless. In the morning, I would go across to the pharmacy and see if they sell Tamoxifen. It is Mexico, you never know unless you ask. The only concern I had, was the quality of the product, and if it indeed was Tamoxifen. It is Mexico, you never know if what you get, is what you ask for. My other plan was to walk around the resort and ask women if they had any spare Tamoxifen. I was able to drift off to sleep for a few more hours, knowing I had some sort of proactive plan.

Not surprisingly, I was up early. I decided to get a coffee and go watch the sun rise on the beach. As I lifted my backpack out of the way, I noticed something that was underneath it on the chair. As soon as my hand touched it, I knew immediately that it was my Tamoxifen card! I couldn't believe my eyes! How did it get there? We both looked through the backpack and all around. It didn't matter, I let out an emphatic "yes" with a fist pump, and did a little happy dance! I was happy and relieved. In my excitement, Cheryl rolled over and asked what was going on. As I flashed her the familiar blue card, she too smiled and giggled in excitement. As it turned out she too woke up a few times through the night trying to figure out solutions to my Tamoxifen issue. Clearly, the importance of this drug impacts more than just me. Keeping my system in its new "unbalanced balance", and the cancer away, is a family affair.

Here is what I know to be true about Tamoxifen. While it has chemically altered my hormones and my body, as I know it, it is also the best chance I have at keeping my estrogen dominate cancer from coming back. There are women everywhere, who are facing advanced stages of breast cancer and would do anything to be Stage II and taking Tamoxifen. When I shift my perspective and consider both sides of the coin, I recognize that I am pretty blessed to be where I am at, as healthy as I am.

March 4 will mark three years that I have been taking Tamoxifen. Two years ago I did ask the Oncologist why the standard dosing time went from five years to ten, to which he replied, "Studies show less of a chance of recurrence if patients stay on it for ten years, so that is the new standard." To which I then asked, what happens at the ten year mark? Do the cancer cells say, "Hey, good for you. You made it ten years, so as your reward for taking this drug, we are just going to leave you alone now. Take care and have a great rest of your life."

The Oncologist smiled in amusement and said, "Unfortunately, it's not that easy. My guess is by the time you are at the ten-year mark, the standard will be for life."

I don't really want to go into a lot of details right now, as to what I experienced with Tamoxifen. Every woman is different and will respond differently to it. I don't want to cause alarm or negatively influence your experience before you even have a chance to see how your body responds.

If you gain a clear understanding of what menopause is and prepare yourself for those possible side effects, you will feel in better control than if you hop on an Internet chat forum and get lost down a rabbit hole of misinformation and heated emotions.

Whatever hormone therapy you end up on, know that you will have an adjustment period. My adjustment time took about 2.5 years, before I began to feel more in balance. Those thirty months were a struggle, but I never gave up on myself. It would have been easier to throw in the towel, eat the cake and let my body go, but I knew that wasn't who I was. I, Cindy, am a strong, fit, healthy, vibrant woman. I am a source of strength from which to impact the world. I knew what my level of healthy was and I was determined to find it again.

Believe in yourself and know that slow and steady wins this race.

CHAPTER 4:

Radiation—Leg Four of the Climb

Big Picture Processing Questions

Please take a moment to ask yourself these Big Picture Processing questions.

- **What two words describe how I feel right now?**

- **What is the worst-case scenario? What will my life look like if I have to travel down this road?**

- **What is the best-case scenario? What will my life look like if I have to travel down this road?**

- **Who do I want to be in relation to what I am experiencing here and now?**

- **What am I grateful for?**

I touched a little bit on radiation in my round three and four of the chemo chapters.

What two words describe how I feel right now? Tired and anxious.

What is the worst-case scenario? That my skin gets burnt really bad or I get lymphedema. **What will my life look like if I have to travel down this road?** Devastating. It will be an entirely new journey to climb through.

What is the best-case scenario? That my skin and tissues heal well from the burns, and I get back to my pre-treatment strength and mobility. **What will my life look like if I have to**

travel down this road? It might take a while but overall, I will feel like nothing has changed.

Who do I want to be in relation to what I am experiencing here and now? I am a strong, fit, healthy woman. I will crest this mountain knowing I did everything I could to slay this beast.

What am I grateful for? That cancer treatment has become so specific and individualized. While protocol may be the same, each person is looked at and treated based on their specific cancer.

I remember my first radiation session like it was yesterday. I changed into my gown and they led me down a tunnel, quite similar to the runway you walk down when getting on a plane. Except instead of being greeted by flight attendants, I was greeted by radiation technicians. I have to say, it did feel a little wrong heading into a tunnel that has a huge warning sign and flashing lights that say, "Do not enter, danger, radiation."

The rad techs were fantastic at greeting me, setting me up, and giving me direction throughout each session. Even though I was by myself in the room, hearing their voices over the intercom helped me feel not so alone.

Like chemotherapy, radiation isn't just a one size fits all approach. Your type of breast cancer, staging and if you had surgery or not, all play a factor in whether radiation will be a part of your treatment plan or not. For example, I met some women who had 20-25 radiation sessions, while others like myself had 16. I met other women, who didn't have any radiation. The other thing I should mention is that for some women, radiation is introduced before chemotherapy, while others like myself, had it after. Your oncologist and radiologist will work together to determine the best plan for you.

The radiation appointments are pretty fast. It took me longer to get there and get ready than the actual session itself. The first 10 sessions seemed pretty uneventful. It was during the last 6, that I could tell my tissues were starting to protest. My chest was getting quite pink and hot from the inside out. It reminded me of heating up something in the microwave. While the surface seems somewhat cool, the inside is sizzling.

As my tissues began to deteriorate from the radiation, I did my best to keep my arm mobile. I noticed that even with exercises, my chest and arm were starting to feel tighter and restricted. I was concerned about getting lymphedema, as it was a possible side-effect. I remember doing BPP, as I was feeling some hard-core fear around getting lymphedema. BPP around Lymphedema

What two words describe how I feel right now? Nervous and no control.

What is the worst-case scenario? I get Lymphedema, and it doesn't go away. **What will my life look like if I have to travel down this road?** It will change. While my breasts were a part of me, they didn't change how my body moved or functioned. It changed the way I looked, but I could still do life quite normally. With lymphedema, that will open a whole different can of worms.

What is the best-case scenario? That I get through my treatment and healing without any lymphedema. **What will my life look like if I have to travel down this road?** Nothing will change. I will continue doing what I can to help my body heal.

Who do I want to be in relation to what I am experiencing here and now? I know I can't control if I get lymphedema or not. The only thing I can control is how I choose to respond to it. I choose to respond to it with a warrior mindset. I will look fear in the eye and rise above it.

What am I grateful for? That radiation treatment will increase my survival rate. While lymphedema can happen, it really is just a small chance. I won't waste anymore precious time worrying about something that may or may not happen.

I knew I was getting close to the summit and focused all my energy on getting to the top!

Journal Entry:

Easter Wishes and Update

March 18, 2016

Good afternoon,

I am very happy to report, I am halfway through radiation! (Yay!)

The technology and advancements for radiation treatment is quite remarkable. Every day I ask questions and learn more about the process. I have to say, I am impressed by how individualized and specific the treatment is. I have absolute full confidence in my doctor, the process and the wonderful radiation techs who administer the treatment.

Because it was my left side that had the cancer, it is my left side that gets radiation. I am starting to turn a beautiful shade of pink. So far my skin feels like a sunburn, except along my incision, it is getting really sore and tender. I have to laugh because when looking at my burn pattern, the left half of my torso has taken on the shape of the Alberta province!

Overall, I would say radiation is way easier than chemo! The biggest thing, aside from the burnt skin is fatigue. It, combined with the compounding chemo fatigue, definitely has my number. I am doing daily exercises and stretching to keep my energy moving and to keep my skin, muscles and joints from adhering. So far so good!

On a super positive note... Spring has sprung and so is my hair!

I have been sporting a skin head for three months and I have to say, losing my hair really didn't faze me. I chose to embrace it and enjoy some of the advantages of being bald. For instance;

- Getting showered and dressed is fast. So very fast!

- No toque or hat head.

- No bed head.

- Saved money on highlights and haircuts.

- Saved money on shampoo.

- No bad hair days.

- Being able to enjoy the feel of soft smooth skin.

Just this week my hair has begun to poke through. I took a picture, but you can't really see anything yet. I guess at this stage it's more of a 'feel' thing. AND it feels great! Prickly, but great!

That is it for now. I will see you, in a couple of weeks, at the top, for the next update!

Thank you for your love and support. I wish you and your families a wonderful Easter!

CHAPTER 5:

The Summit—Leg Five of the Climb

The Final Treatment

Big Picture Processing Questions

Please take a moment to ask yourself these Big Picture Processing questions.

- **What two words describe how I feel right now?**

- **What is the worst-case scenario? What will my life look like if I have to travel down this road?**

- **What is the best-case scenario? What will my life look like if I have to travel down this road?**

- **Who do I want to be in relation to what I am experiencing here and now?**

- **What am I grateful for?**

Here is my blog from when I reached that summit, that captures my BPP:

Journal Entry: Top of the Mountain
April 5, 2016

Today is a day to remember. I feel blessed in so many ways, I almost don't know where to begin.

I completed the last treatment, of my final step, and am now standing on top of my cancer mountain. I am DONE!

As I reflect back on this eight-month journey, I am amazed at what I have been through. Since my slap of reality biopsy back on Aug 26, I have had my spiritual warrior out, and my game face on. Through the blood, sweat (even more now with this instant menopause), and tears, Cheryl and I have climbed a very steep, challenging and rough mountain. It tried to chew me up and spit me out a few times, but I stood my ground! I had my eyes on the top and there was no stopping me.

Every good climber is only as good as their equipment and support team. I am so blessed and fortunate to have had amazing treatment and care from the doctors, nurses and support staff here in Red Deer. Right from my double mastectomy, through chemo, (and all of its side show shenanigans), and finishing off with a tan of a lifetime in radiation. I am confident that because of the grunt work and discomfort of the last six months, I am going to live a long and healthy life.

A long, healthy life would be empty without friends and family. Throughout this entire process, I have had 360 degrees of support, that cheered and encouraged me along, and up that mountain. Cheryl and I have been continually blown away by your generosity and love.

Today, on my last day of climbing, I received a helping of love and support that will keep my heart and soul full for decades to come.

As I came out of the radiation hallway, I was greeted by Cheryl, who had a big smile on her face, tears in her eyes and holding a bottle of Dom Perignon Champagne. As I came out of the hallway, I was met by a semi-circle of cheering, laughing and crying friends, who gathered to celebrate my top of the mountain moment.

Cheryl managed to organize a group of 14 friends to arrive at the hospital between 8:05 a.m. and 8:10 a.m. to surprise me and witness the end of my climb. It wasn't just me on this climb. Cancer is a journey that impacts family and friends in ways the climber will never know. I am blessed that Cheryl put together a moment for everyone to celebrate.

Thank you all for your hugs, laughter and tears!

What is it with the Dom Perignon? Well, a week after my surgery, I was lying in bed one sleepless night watching a movie where the couple was drinking Dom. The Maitre D says to the couple, "What did Dom Perignon say to fellow monks after he invented champagne?

Come quickly, I am tasting the stars." I love stars! I decided right then and there it would be a shame if I went through my life and never tasted Dom Perignon. The next day I told Cheryl that when I am through treatment, I am buying myself some Dom Perignon. As you read above, Cheryl surprised me with a bottle this morning.

So what is next? RECOVERY! Even though radiation is done, apparently my tissues will continue to "cook" for another ten days and may crack and blister. I am emotionally, mentally and physically exhausted. This girl needs to recharge her batteries big time. Eight months of stress and poison takes a toll. The best way I can explain my energy... Remember back in the days of listening to a tape in a walkman, and as the batteries start to die, the song slows down and the words get slurred? That is what happens to me. I am going along, I slow down, get mentally confused, slur a bit and then need a rest. This spiritual warrior is ready to recharge and get her vitality back. Let the second half of the journey begin.

Thank you all for your continued love and support.

Journal Entry: After The Summit
May 2, 2016

I reached the top of my cancer mountain on April 5, 2016. I was physically and mentally exhausted as I stood on that peak. I raised my arms in victory knowing I just finished six months of intense treatment. I was done! It was time to catch my breath and get down from this beast of a mountain!

Up until now, I had been picturing this journey as an up and down mountain. The climb straight up, fierce and exhausting. The top, a brief stay with enough time to celebrate and rest up. Then coming down would be straight and steady.

I pictured the descent to be fairly easy, especially compared to the ugly conditions and obstacles I had to deal with on the climb up. I figured because I am a strong, fit and healthy person, I would gain back my vitality pretty quick, and be back on level ground in no time.

I am beginning to see that the landscape isn't quite what I pictured. Instead of the up and down of a single mountain, it is actually a straight up peak, and to get back down, I need to do a little scrambling over a mountain range before I am finished.

The reason for my change in perception? Well, now that I have made it to the top, I am able to see that getting down from this cancer peak isn't as easy and clear cut as I originally thought. There really isn't a path to follow.

On the way up, I was given a destination, directions, trail descriptions, and a pretty accurate timeline of each leg of the climb. Coming down this mountain, is all up to me. Because every climber going through cancer is so different, only I can know when I feel healthy and back to normal. I am my own guide!

The only thing I have been told, is that "Your body will need time to heal, and the timeframe is generally equal to the amount of treatment time. You will experience fatigue. Listen to your body. You will experience side effects with the Tamoxifen, most likely hot flashes. Give it some time, and if you are having trouble sleeping, we can give you something for that. Good luck. If you have any problems, contact us."

To be clear, there is support from different departments at the cancer centre. There is nutrition, self esteem, physiotherapy and occupational therapy available. With my background in personal development, exercise, health and wellness, I have those bases covered. I feel confident I can get myself down the mountain and regain full strength, health and vitality. It might be at a slower pace than I want, but part of this journey is learning to take one step at a time and accept what is. For example, my old ways of doing things and pushing my limits, is not working for me right now. I am learning quickly, there is a fine line between a 'proactive, just try it' push and a 'I over did it, now I'm sidelined' push.

My new body, enjoys movement, stretching and light resistance. But shuts down quickly if I overdo anything. In fact, my system is so sensitive right now, that excess stimuli of anything, good or bad, turns to stress and shuts me down. Learning what my body defines as "excess" is important, so I can modify what I'm doing to help keep my feet moving forward.

What does a shut-down feel like? My body gets that internal shaking, as though I am having a blood sugar crash. My eyes and ears feel like they are filling with pressure and want to explode. My eyelids want to close and shut off all stimuli. My breathing becomes labored, and if I don't rest immediately when I feel these symptoms, nausea will take over. I recently learned that if I push through and ignore these symptoms, I will be exhausted and depleted, and end up needing bed rest, which then puts me behind in the healing process.

While I'm not happy with this new response system of mine, I accept that, it is what it is, and I, at least know and understand it has hot buttons and limits. This knowledge will help me define a level of health for my "new" normal and strategize a program that will support it.

I'm hoping that once my energy gets flowing and I can get consistent with exercise, it will help me adapt to the crazy hormone changes and sleep deprivation Tamoxifen has created. This will be a bit of an uphill battle, but I am confident that with dedicated focus over the next few months, I will recapture my strength, health and vitality, get back to work, be down this mountain, done with this journey and live happily ever after!

I still have some peaks, distance, and work to do before I am done with this cancer journey.

Recovering from Battle

Fighting breast cancer is a fierce battle. You will be challenged not just physically, but mentally, emotionally, and spiritually all at the same time. Now more than ever, you need to rediscover and embrace your inner warrior so you can be in control of what is left of your precious time, no matter how long that may be.

I believe that you are here on Earth to experientially learn who you are by every time/space event you encounter, including big ugly ones called Cancer. I also believe that no matter what stage of cancer you are diagnosed with, you can choose to thrive your climb. Thrive doesn't mean everything is sunshine and roses, it means that you have decided to stand tall, look fear in the eye and continue to learn, grow and create yourself anew in every moment, of everyday, until your last breath.

I know that for some women, especially those diagnosed with Stage IV breast cancer, the reference to being a Warrior can feel a bit cliché. I know that when you are given a terminal diagnosis, you may feel that the battle is almost over, so why fight? Why put in the time and effort to make changes now, when the end is so near? Why start climbing a bitch of a mountain when the chances of you reaching the top are slim?

I say you fight for the same reasons as someone diagnosed with stage 0-III would. From your hardest struggles, you often learn your biggest lessons, get your greatest questions answered, and you may even find that inner peace you have been searching for your entire life. You are now facing a climb that will challenge you on every level of your being. You want to be dialed into your inner warrior, so, no matter how many steps you are left with, you are choosing to come from a place of personal power and intention.

To be clear, fighting cancer doesn't mean resisting what is, it means that you are going to put all your effort into experiencing the bigger picture, getting the ultimate lesson, or perhaps understanding what your true purpose in life is. You fight to keep your feet moving forward. You fight to keep your Warrior Mindset. You fight so when it's over, you know that you showed up for yourself. That my friend, is worth the hype of pulling up your big girl panties and getting your game face on. It is time you rediscover and embrace your inner warrior so you can climb this Pink Mountain and seize whatever learning opportunities are ahead of you.

Wherever you go from here, wherever the next steps on your journey take you, I encourage you to continue exploring your life from a shifted perspective. Your life is an amazing experience designed just for you, and when you choose to consciously participate, you are choosing to live in a state of empowerment. You are choosing to pick up the pieces of the puzzle and are choosing to understand your soul's purpose.

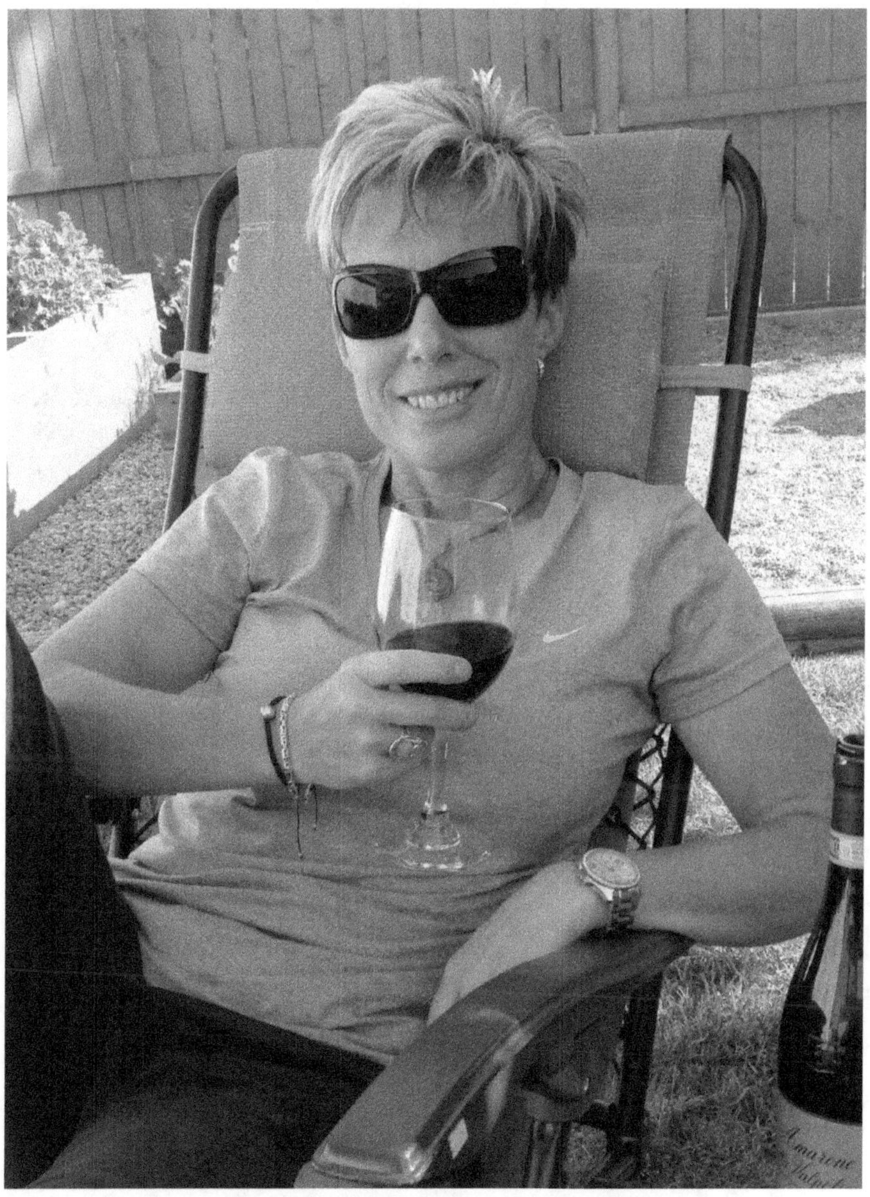

45th Birthday

One week before the mammogram that changed everything

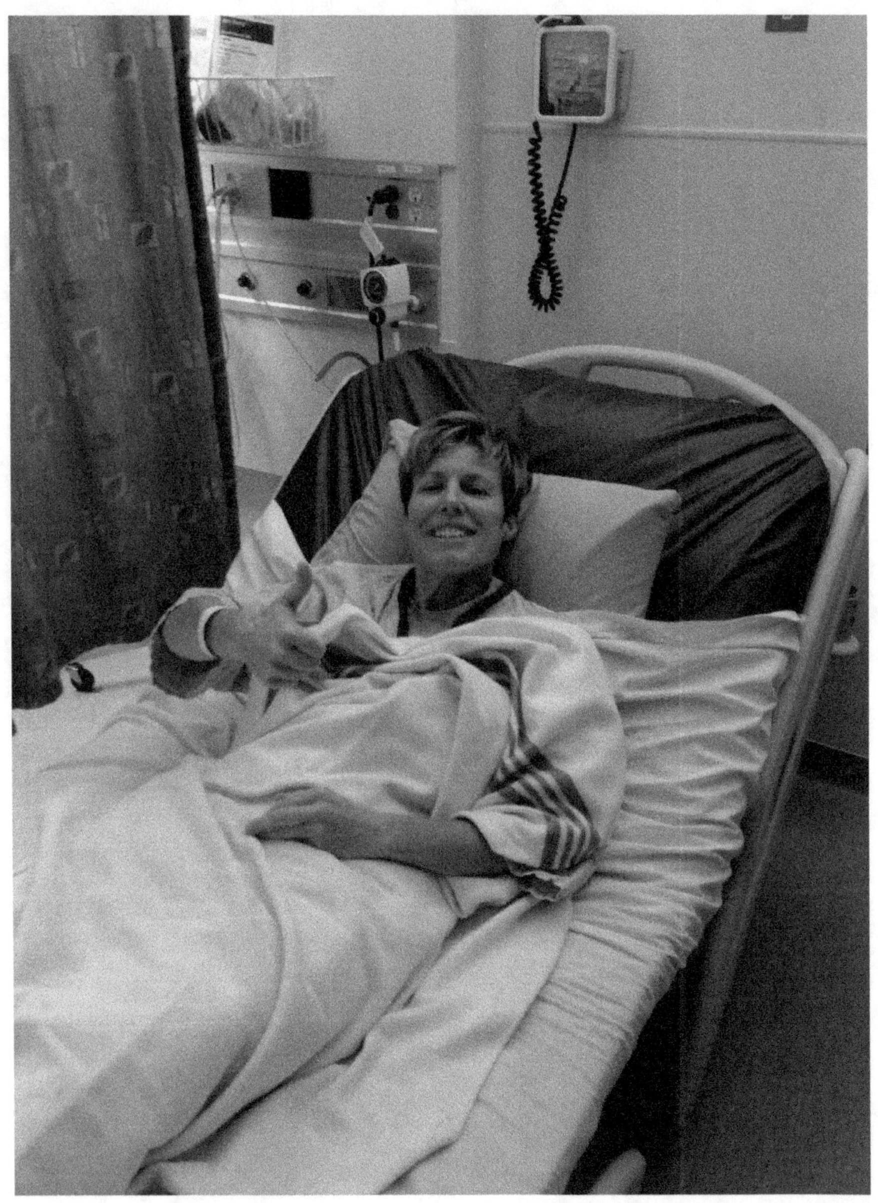

Before my double mastectomy surgery

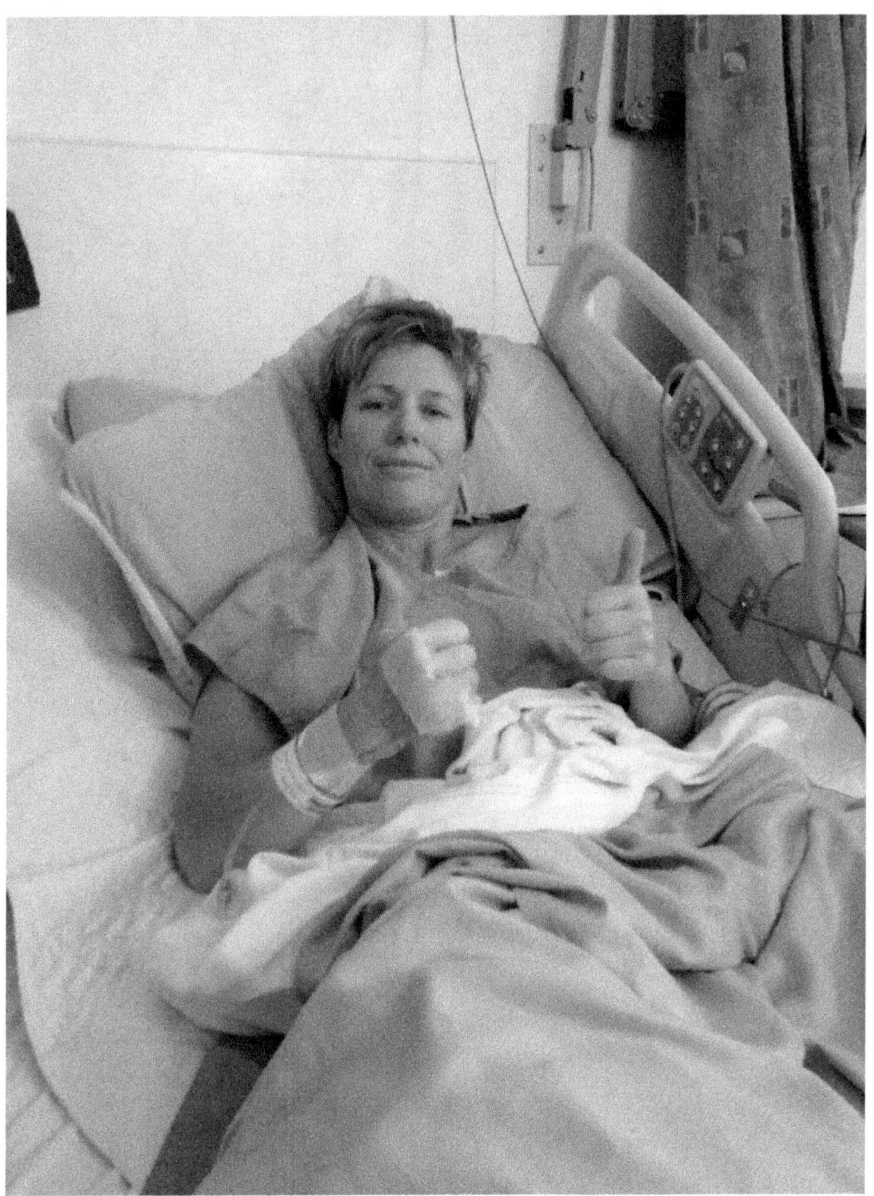

After Surgery

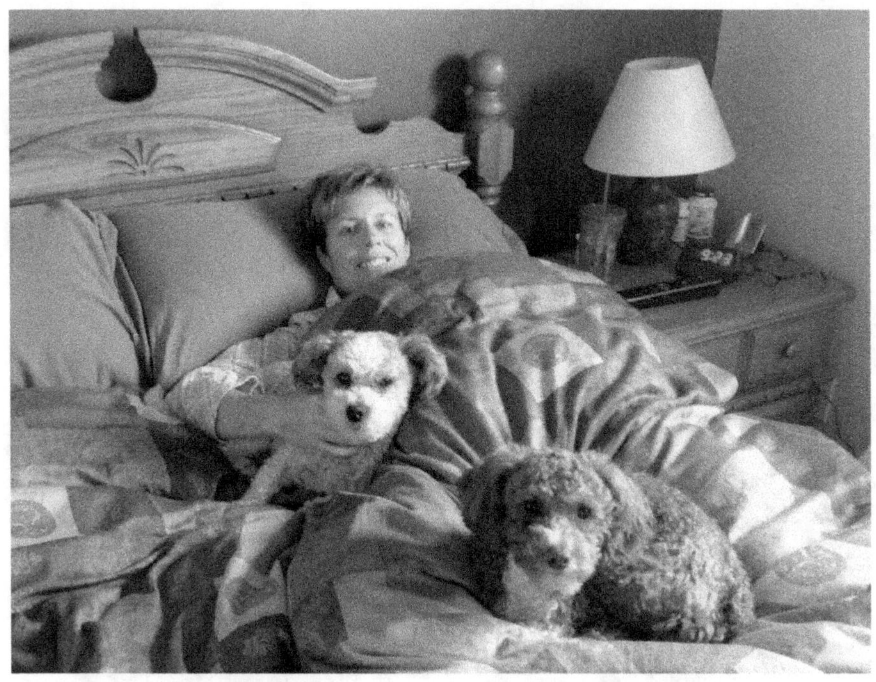

Always feeling the love with Rusty and Ringo

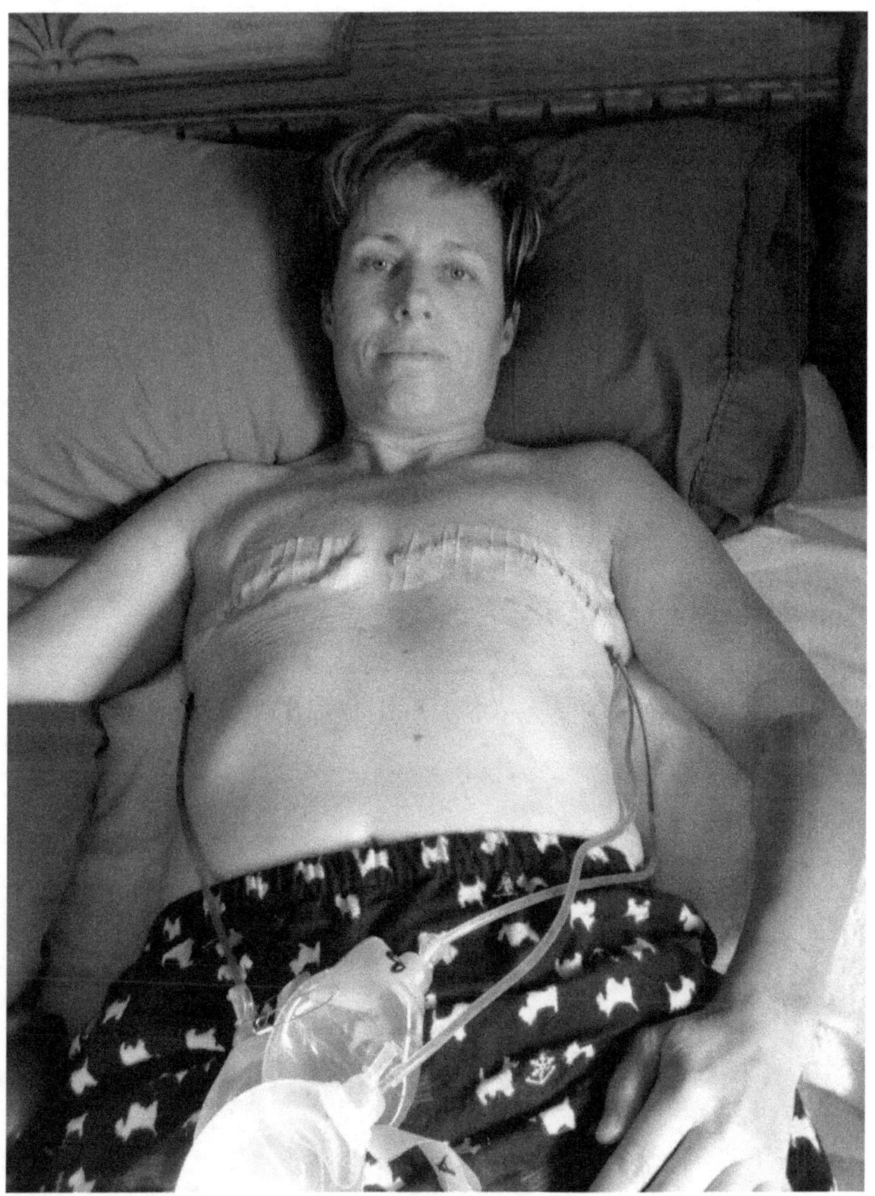

Seeing my chest for the first time

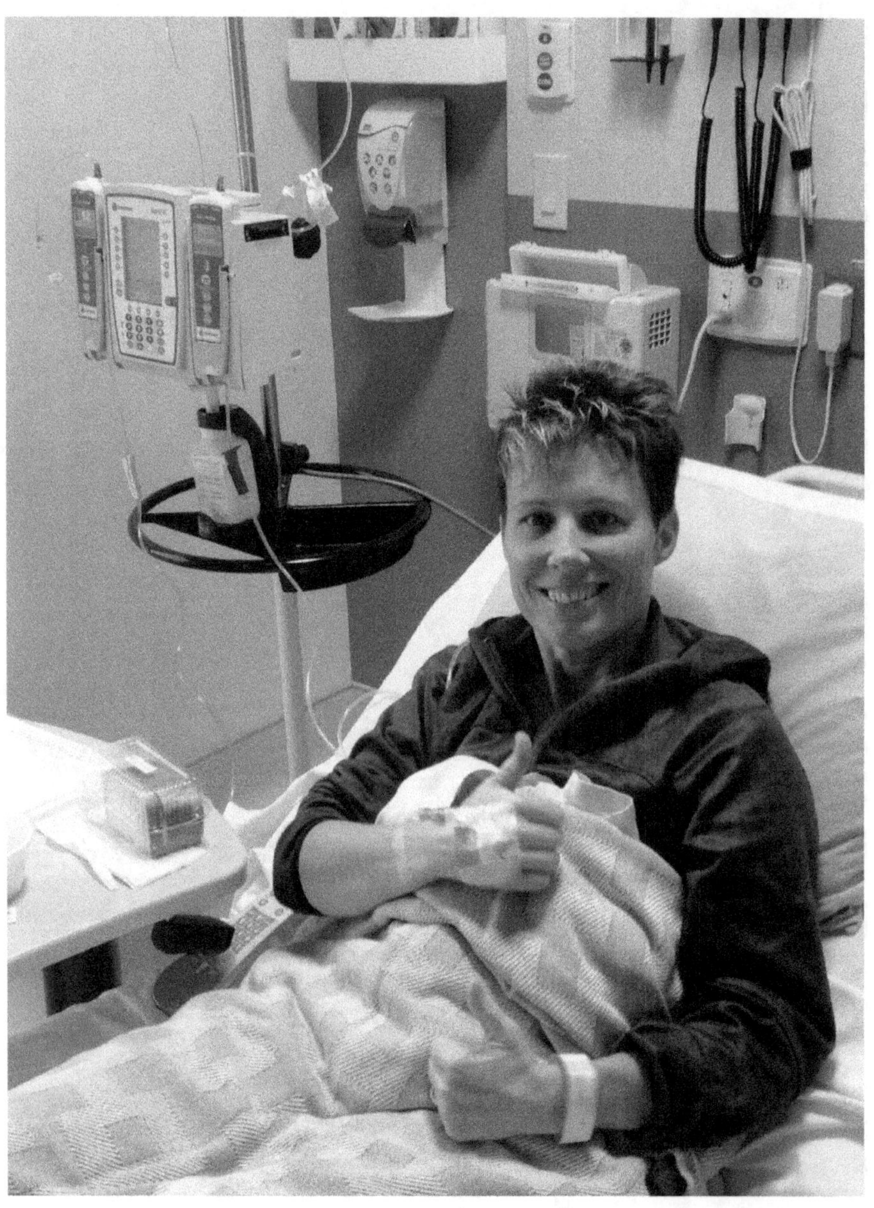

First round of chemo

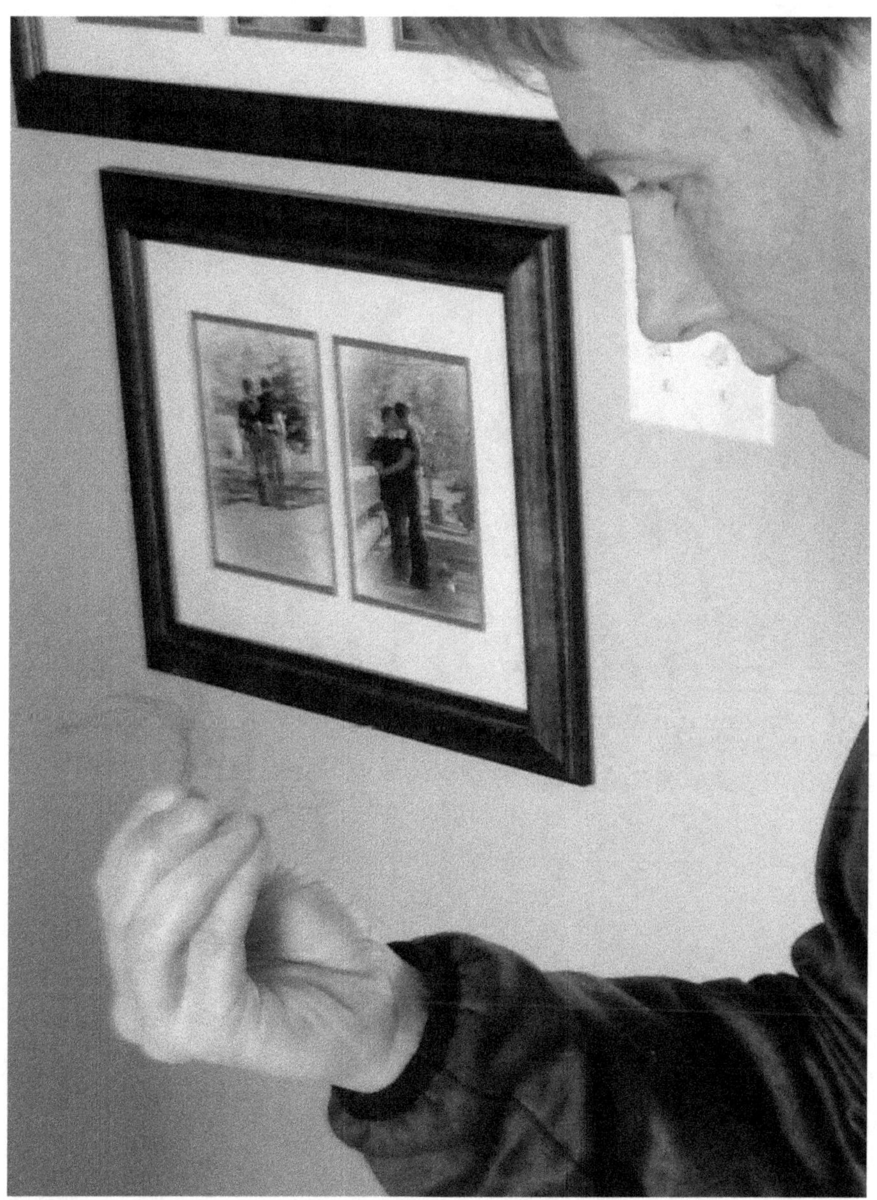

Losing my hair

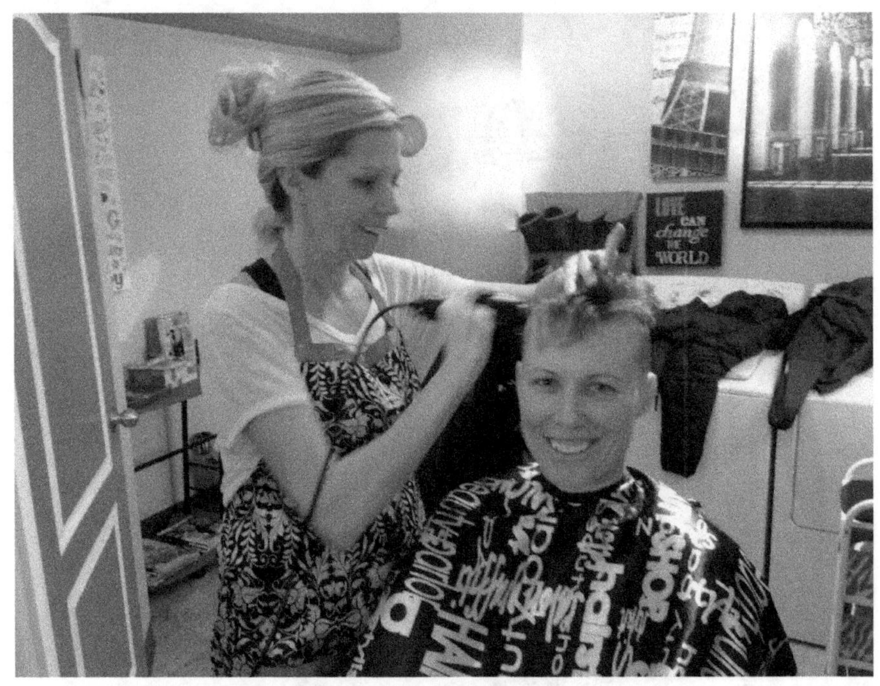

Having fun as my friend Tanya gives me a G.I. Jane look

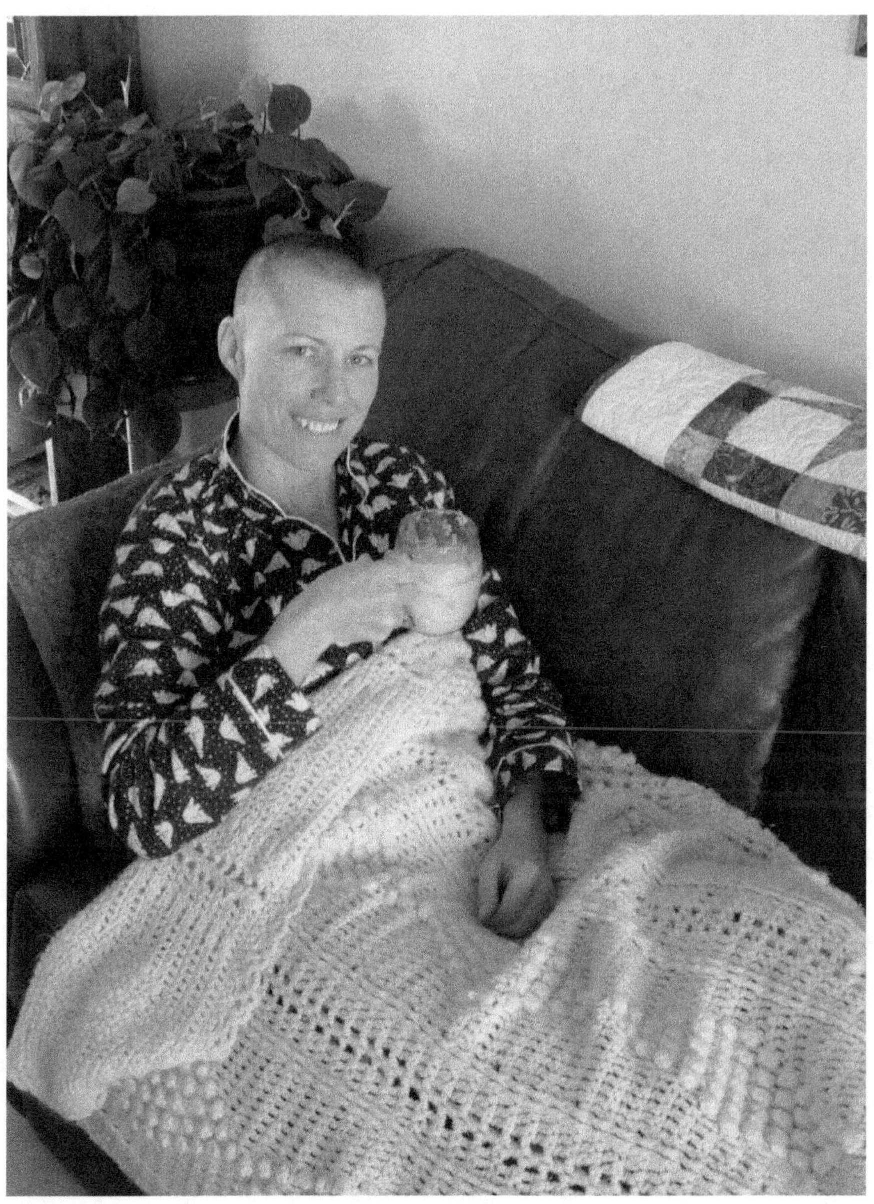

Christmas morning

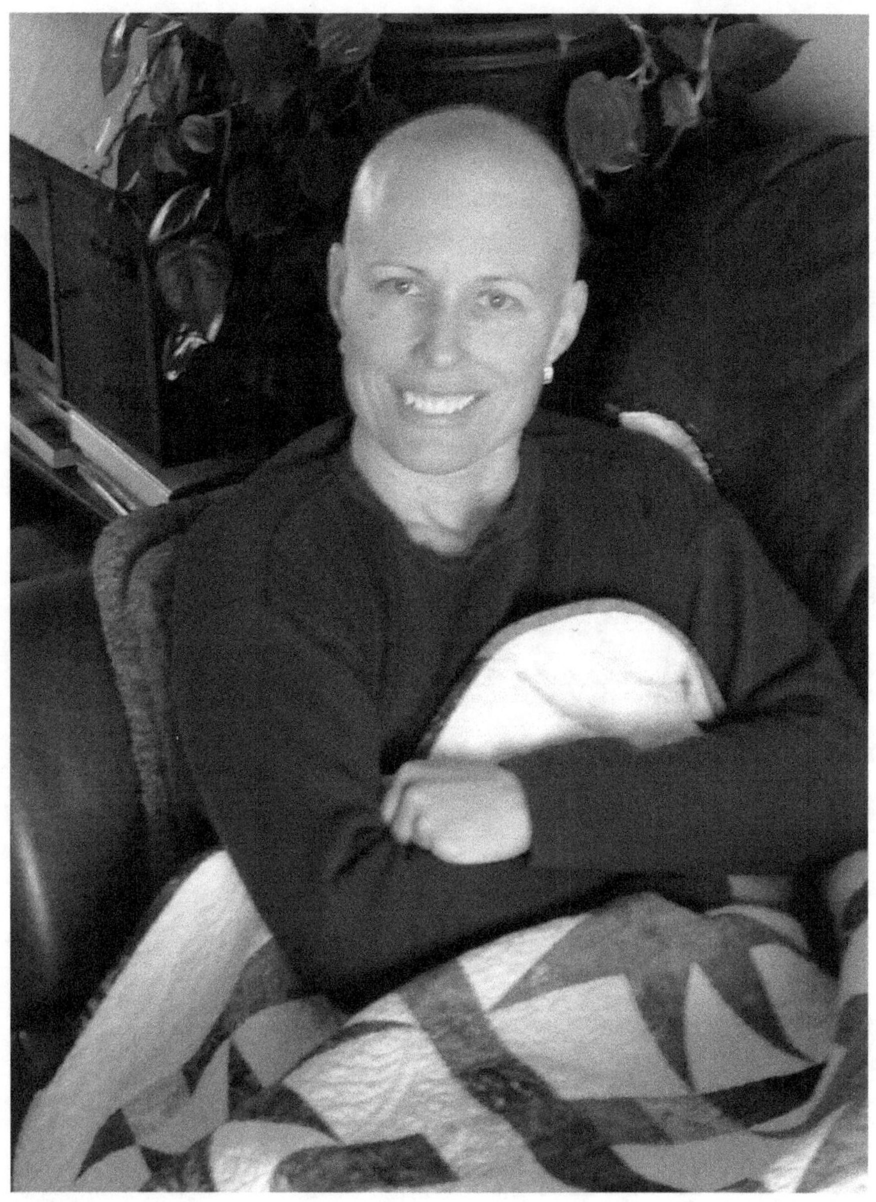

First time completely bald

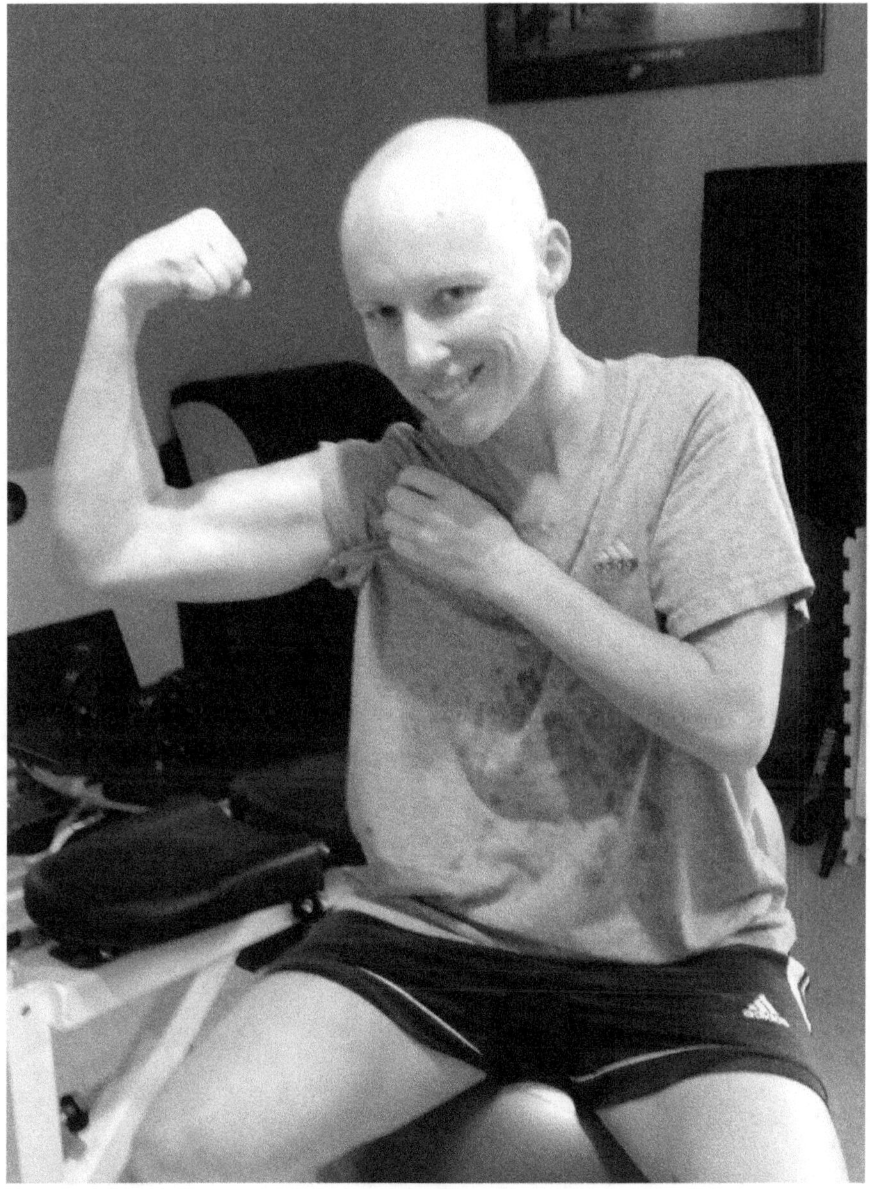

Keeping my exercise up. Before the ass kicking of another round of chemo

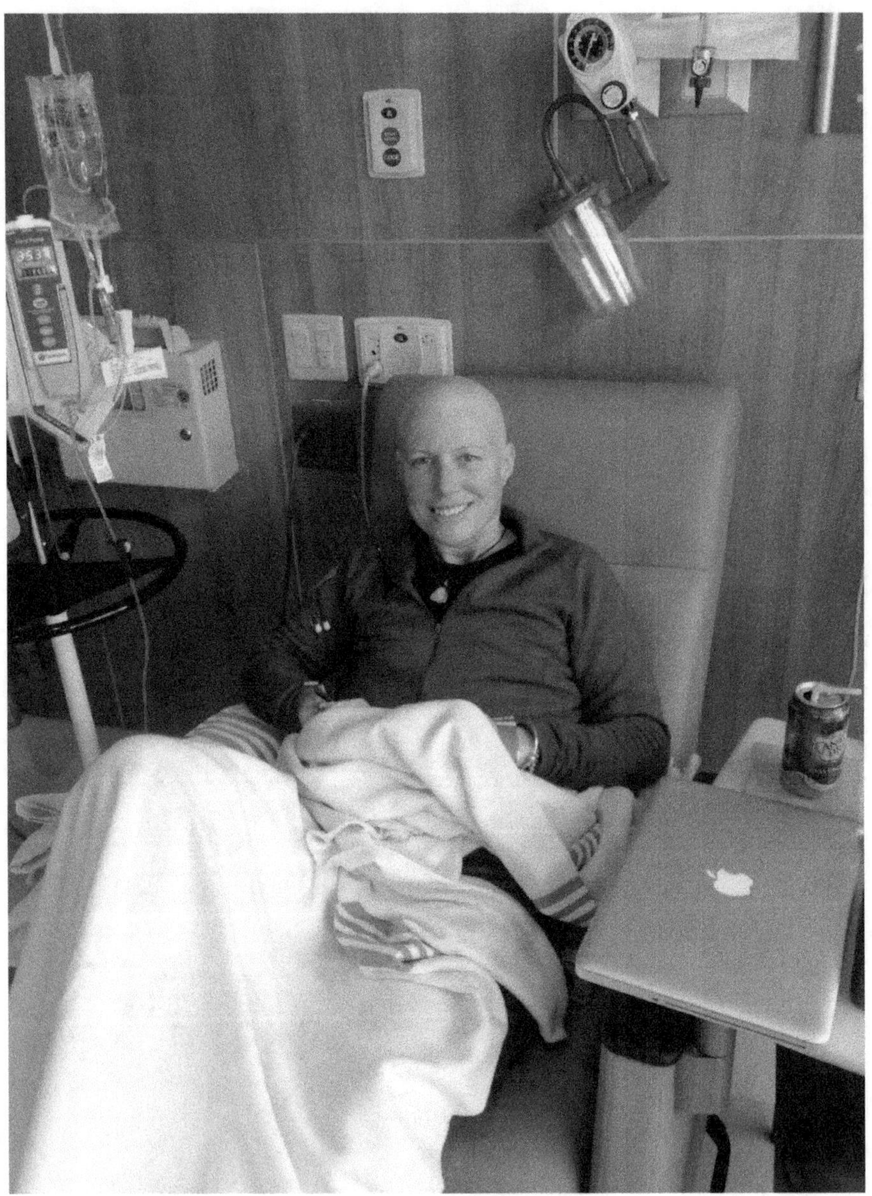

Last round of chemo

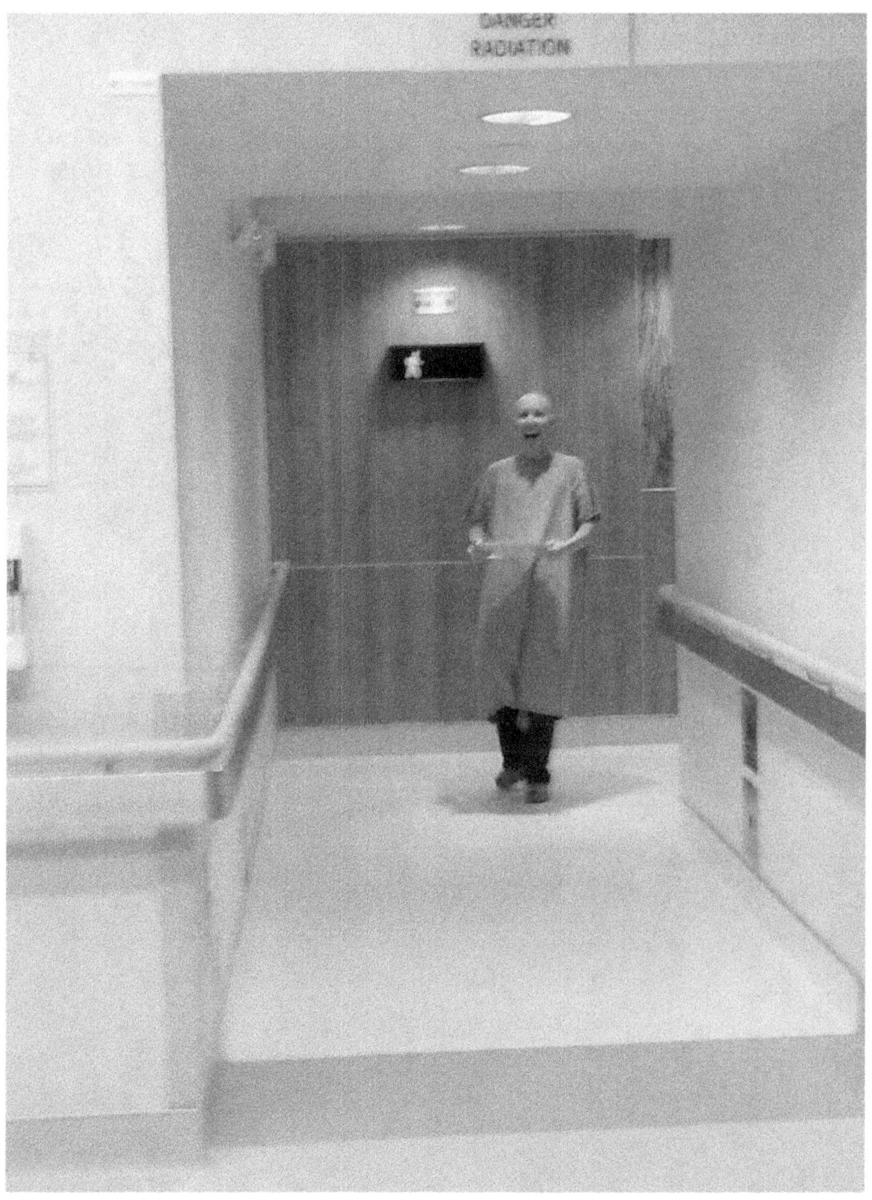

Coming out of the radiation tunnel for the last time,

to a surprise party

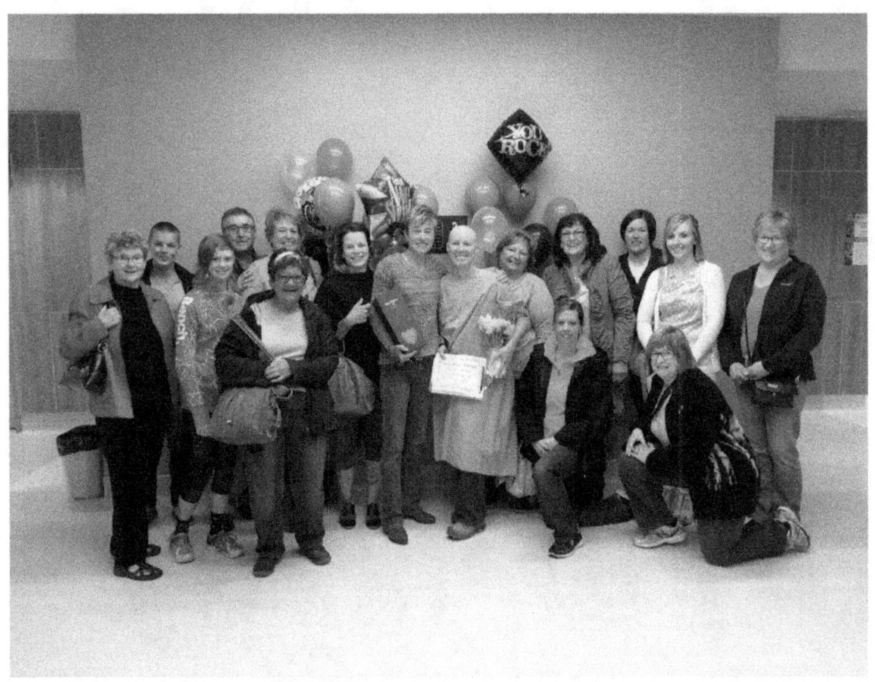

A moment at the top of the mountain with friends

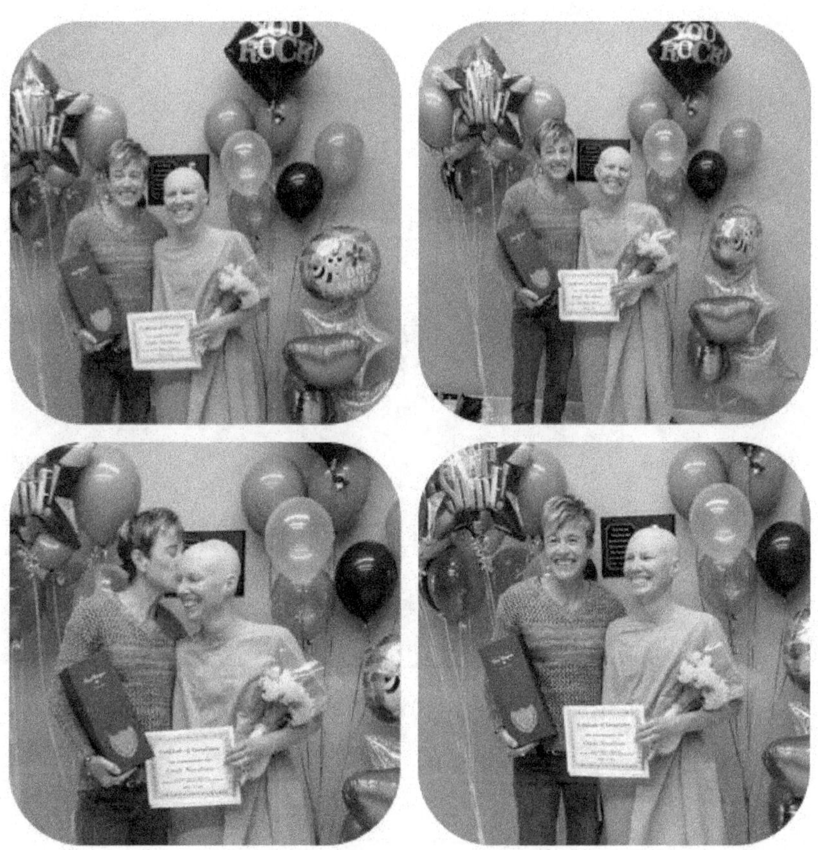

Cheryl and I made it. We got through cancer treatment

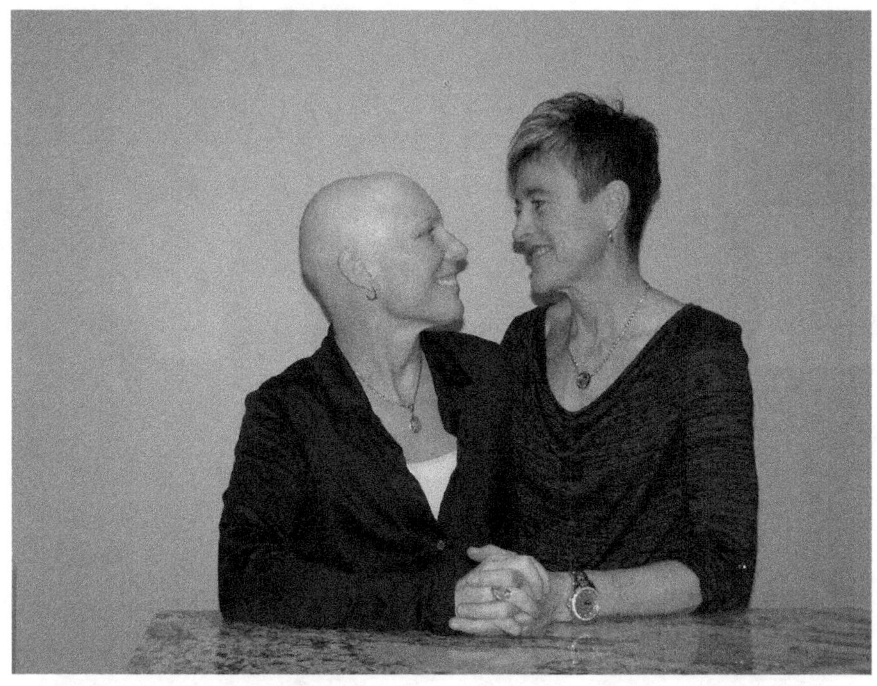

My best friend and my rock…my partner of 20 years, Cheryl

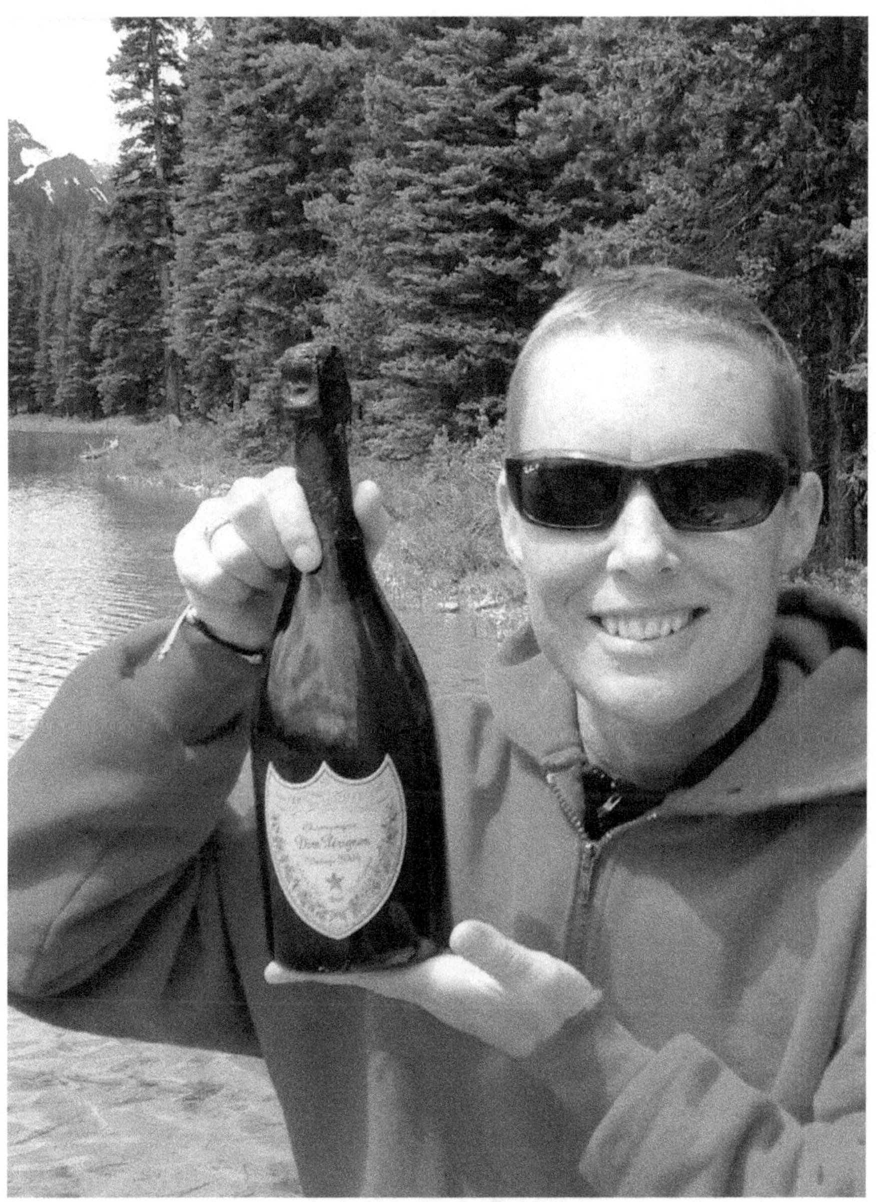

Enjoying the Dom Perignon,

a couple months later in the mountains!

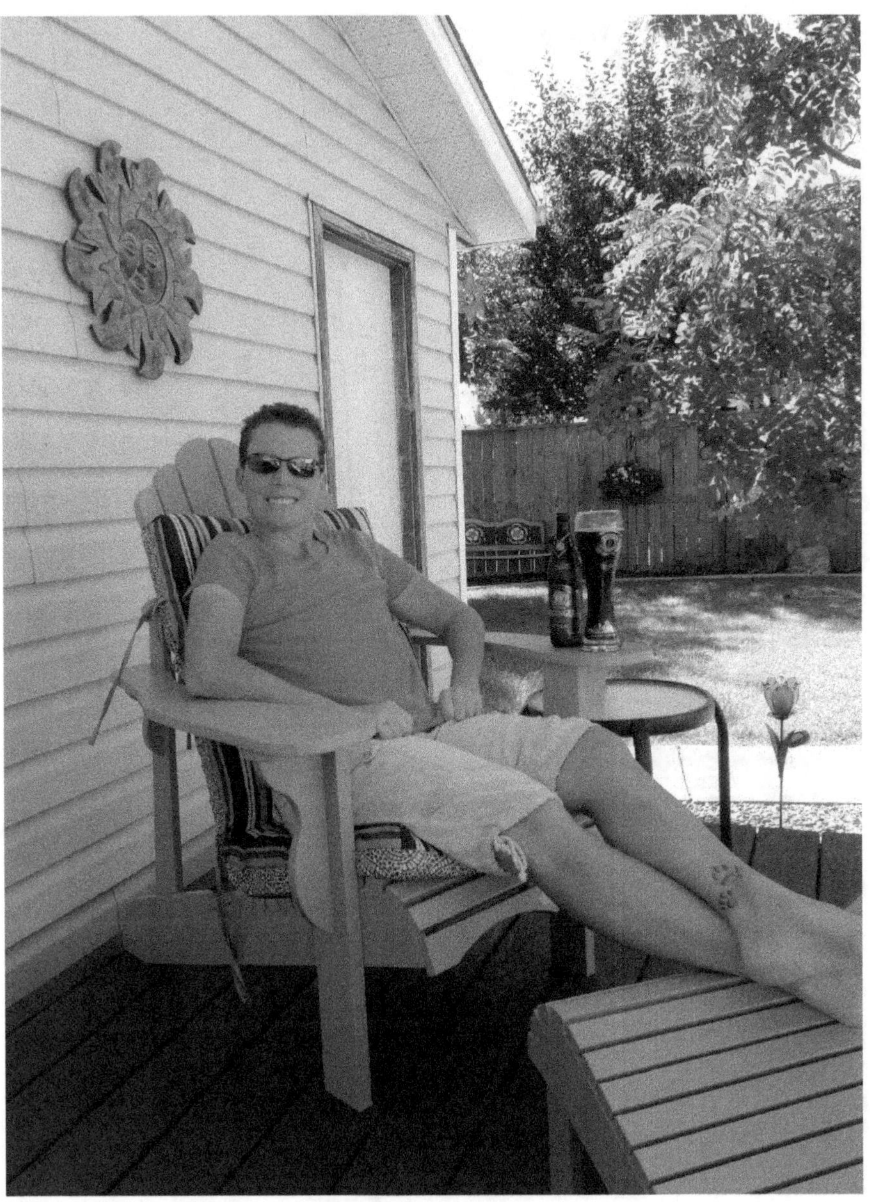

Celebrating my 46th birthday

Resources

Thank you for picking up and making this book a part of your life as you climb the pink mountain.

I've been where you are and understand the range of emotions that can overtake your mind, body and spirit throughout this journey. For that reason, I encourage you to keep this book handy so you can refer back to it. Reading and nodding your head to the ideas and concepts laid out in this book is one level of learning. As a breast cancer patient who wants to stay out of fear, anger, or the risk of spiralling out of control, you are choosing to take different actions. You have the power right now to choose a different path.

It's for that reason that I created a companion workbook called, Empower Your Climb. It is a full-blown mindset workbook, that will help you become aware of your blocks and keep your feet moving forward, as you make your way up the pink mountain.

Get the Empower Your Climb Companion Workbook here:

www.thrivetheclimb.com/companion-workbook

You are not alone on this journey. It is my vision and mission to help you rediscover your inner warrior so you can thrive your climb.

When you find the inner light of your spirit,

you find your true potential and power!

About the Author

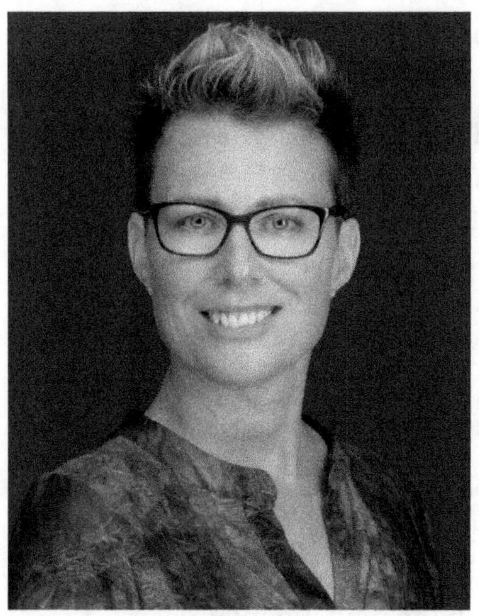

Cindy Needham, Breast Cancer Warrior/Mindset Mentor, has committed her life to applying a spirit-based, warrior mindset to life's many challenges. Cindy has toiled to unravel the enigma of how physical and spiritual wellness are entangled through extensive education and research. Over the past 30 years, she has developed a methodology to experience life with a higher level of consciousness and purpose.

Rivalling many obstacles in her life, she met her lifetime challenger of —climbing The Pink Mountain—when she was diagnosed with breast cancer. Using the arsenal of skills, she curated from previous triumphs, she faced her Pink Mountain as a warrior. Cindy chronicled her personal journey using these techniques with the mission of empowering other women facing a similar battle.

Supporting women going through breast cancer is what Cindy does. Inspiring them to shift their perspective and tap into their inner strength beyond their imagination, is who she is.